Lecture Notes in Computer Science   10170

Commenced Publication in 1973
Founding and Former Series Editors:
Gerhard Goos, Juris Hartmanis, and Jan van Leeuwen

Terry Peters · Guang-Zhong Yang
Nassir Navab · Kensaku Mori
Xiongbiao Luo · Tobias Reichl
Jonathan McLeod (Eds.)

Computer-Assisted and Robotic Endoscopy

Third International Workshop, CARE 2016
Held in Conjunction with MICCAI 2016
Athens, Greece, October 17, 2016
Revised Selected Papers

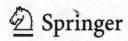

Springer

Editors
Terry Peters
Robarts Research Institute
London, ON
Canada

Guang-Zhong Yang
Imperial College London
London
UK

Nassir Navab
Johns Hopkins University
Baltimore, MD
USA

Kensaku Mori
Graduate School of Information Science
Nagoya University
Nagoya
Japan

Xiongbiao Luo
Department of Computer Science
Xiamen University
Xiamen
China

Tobias Reichl
KUKA Robotics
Augsburg, Bayern
Germany

Jonathan McLeod
Robarts Research Institute
Western University
London
Canada

ISSN 0302-9743   ISSN 1611-3349   (electronic)
Lecture Notes in Computer Science
ISBN 978-3-319-54056-6   ISBN 978-3-319-54057-3   (eBook)
DOI 10.1007/978-3-319-54057-3

Library of Congress Control Number: 2017932123

LNCS Sublibrary: SL6 – Image Processing, Computer Vision, Pattern Recognition, and Graphics

Printed on acid-free paper

This Springer imprint is published by Springer Nature
The registered company is Springer International Publishing AG
The registered company address is: Gewerbestrasse 11, 6330 Cham, Switzerland

Preface

Welcome to the proceedings of the third edition of the International Workshop on Computer-Assisted and Robotic Endoscopy (CARE) that was held in conjunction with MICCAI on October 17, 2016, in Athens, Greece.

CARE brings together researchers, clinicians, and medical companies involved in scientific research in the field of computer-assisted and robotic endoscopy to advance current endoscopic medical interventions. The next generation of CARE systems promises to integrate multimodal information relative to the patient's anatomy, the control status of medical endoscopes and surgical tools, and the actions of surgical staff to guide endoscopic interventions. To this end, technical advances should be introduced in many areas, such as computer vision, graphics, robotics, medical imaging, external tracking systems, medical device controls systems, information processing techniques, endoscopy planning and simulation.

The technical program of this workshop comprised original and high-quality papers that, together with this year's keynotes, explored the most recent scientific, technological, and translational advancements and challenges toward the next generation of CARE systems. We selected 11 high-quality papers from nine countries this year. All the selected papers were revised and resubmitted by the authors in accordance with the reviewers' comments and the volume editors' suggestions.

It was also our great honor and pleasure to welcome the keynote speakers, Dr. Pierre Jannin (INSERM and University of Rennes 1), Prof. Dr. Nassir Navab (Johns Hopkins University, USA), and Dr. Mahdi Azizian (Intuitive Surgical Inc., USA), who gave fantastic talks on recent advances in robotic endoscopic interventions from both academic and industrial perspectives.

The CARE 2016 Organizing Committee would like to sincerely thank all Program Committee members for putting their best effort in reviewing all the submissions. We also extend our thanks and appreciation to KUKA Robotics, Germany, for sponsoring the best paper award and Springer for accepting to publish the CARE proceedings in the *Lecture Notes in Computer Science* series. We warmly thank all authors, researcher, and attendees at CARE 2017 for their scientific contribution, enthusiasm, and support. We are looking forward to the continuing support and participation in our next CARE event that will be held in conjunction with MICCAI 2017 in Quebec, Canada.

January 2017

Terry Peters
Guang-Zhong Yang
Nassir Navab
Kensaku Mori
Xiongbiao Luo
Tobias Reichl
Jonathan McLeod

Organization

Organizing Committee

Terry Peters	Western University, Canada
Guang-Zhong Yang	Imperial College London, UK
Nassir Navab	Technische Universität München Germany/JHU, USA
Kensaku Mori	Nagoya University, Japan
Xiongbiao Luo	Xiamen University, China
Tobias Reichl	KUKA Laboratories GmbH, Germany
Jonathan McLeod	Western University, Canada

Program Committee

Andreas Uhl	University of Salzburg, Austria
Austin Reiter	The Johns Hopkins University, USA
Caroline Essert	University of Strasbourg, France
Chaoyang Shi	University of Toronto, Canada
Guoyan Zheng	University of Bern, Switzerland
Holger Roth	National Institutes of Health, USA
Huafeng Wang	Beihang University, China
Jorge Bernal	The Autonomous University of Barcelona, Spain
Kevin Cleary	Children's National Medical Center, USA
Lena Mair-Hein	German Cancer Research Center, Germany
Leo Joskowicz	Hebrew University of Jerusalem, Israel
Mashahiro Oda	Nagoya University, Japan
Menglong Ye	Imperial College London, UK
Paul Loschak	Harvard University, USA
Peter Mountney	Siemens Corporation, UK
Pierre Jannin	University of Rennes 1, France
Pietro Valdastri	Vanderbilt University, USA
Randy Ellis	Queen's University, Canada
Raphael Sznitman	University of Bern, Switzerland
Sebastian Wirkert	German Cancer Research Center, Germany
Siyamalan Manivannan	University of Dundee, UK
Siyang Zuo	Tianjin University, China
Stamatia Giannarou	Imperial College London, UK
Tong Tong	Harvard University, USA
Wei Xiong	A*STAR Institute for Infocomm Research, Singapore
Wenjia Bai	Imperial College London, UK
Xiahai Zhuang	Shanghai Jiaotong University, China
Yoshito Otake	Nara Institute of Science and Technology, Japan

Contents

Transfer Learning for Colonic Polyp Classification Using Off-the-Shelf CNN Features

Eduardo Ribeiro[1,2(✉)], Andreas Uhl[1], Georg Wimmer[1], and Michael Häfner[3]

[1] Department of Computer Sciences, University of Salzburg, Salzburg, Austria
uft.eduardo@uft.edu.br,
uhl@cosy.sbg.ac.at,
gwimmer@cosy.sbg.ac.at
[2] Department of Computer Sciences, Federal University of Tocantins,
Palmas, Tocantins, Brazil
[3] St. Elisabeth Hospital, Vienna, Austria
michael.haefner@elisabethinen-wien.at
http://www.wavelab.at

Abstract. Recently, a great development in image recognition has been achieved, especially by the availability of large and annotated databases and the application of Deep Learning on these data. Convolutional Neural Networks (CNN's) can be used to enable the extraction of highly representative features among the network layers filtering, selecting and using these features in the last fully connected layers for pattern classification. However, CNN training for automatic medical image classification still provides a challenge due to the lack of large and publicly available annotated databases. In this work, we evaluate and analyze the use of CNN's as a general feature descriptor doing transfer learning to generate "off-the-shelf" CNN's features for the colonic polyp classification task. The good results obtained by off-the-shelf CNN's features in many different databases suggest that features learned from CNN with natural images can be highly relevant for colonic polyp classification.

Keywords: Deep learning · Convolutional Neural Networks · Colonic polyp classification

1   Introduction

The leading cause of deaths related to intestinal tract is the development of cancer cells (polyps) in its many parts. An early detection (when the cancer is still at an early stage) can reduce the risk of mortality among these patients. More specifically, colonic polyps (benign tumors or growths which arise on the inner colon surface) have a high occurrence and are known to be precursors of colon cancer development. As a consequence, it is recommended that everyone over an

E. Ribeiro—This research was partially supported by CNPq-Brazil for Eduardo Ribeiro under grant No. 00736/2014-0.

© Springer International Publishing AG 2017
T. Peters et al. (Eds.): CARE 2016, LNCS 10170, pp. 1–13, 2017.
DOI: 10.1007/978-3-319-54057-3_1

age of 50 years be examined regularly [32]. This exam can be done through an endoscopy procedure that is a minimally invasive and relatively painless diagnostic medical procedure that enables specialists to obtain images of internal human body cavities.

Several studies have shown that automatic detection of image regions which may contain polyps within the colon can be used to assist specialists in order to decrease the polyp miss rate [3,28,31]. Such detection can be performed by analyzing the polyp appearance that is generally based on color, shape, texture or spatial features applied to the video frames denoted as polyp detection [1,21,30].

Subsequently, the polyps can be automatically classified using different aspects of shape, color or texture into hyperplastic, adenomatous and malignant. The so-called "pit-pattern" scheme proposed by Kudo et al. [18] can help in diagnosing tumorous lesions once suspicious areas have been detected. In this scheme, the mucosal surface of the colon can be classified into 5 different types designating the size, shape and distribution of the pit structure [6,9,12]. These five pit-pattern types can allow to group the lesions into two main classes: normal mucosa or hyperplastic polyps (healthy class) and neoplastic, adenomatous or carcinomatous structures (abnormal class) as can be seen in Fig. 1(a–d). This approach is quite relevant in clinical practice as shown in a study by Kato et al. [17].

In this work we focus on the polyp classification into these two classes. The different types of pit patterns [18] of these two classes can be observed in Fig. 1(e–f) [14]. However, the classification can be a difficult task due to several factors such as the lack or excess of illumination, the blurring due to movement or water injection and the different appearances of polyps [32]. Also, to find a robust and a global feature extractor that summarizes and represents all these pit-patterns structures in a single vector is very difficult and Deep Learning can be a good alternative to surpass these problems.

Deep learning Neural Networks have been of great interest in recent years, mainly due to the new variations of so-called Convolutional Neural Networks

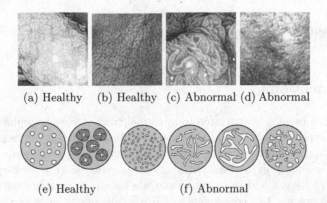

(a) Healthy   (b) Healthy   (c) Abnormal (d) Abnormal

(e) Healthy   (f) Abnormal

Fig. 1. Example images of the two classes (a–d) and the pit-pattern types of these two classes (e–f).

and the use of efficient parallel solvers improved by GPU's [2]. Deep learning is closely related to the high-level representation obtained by raw data such as images and is very effective when applied to large and annotated databases. However, the lack of available annotated medical image databases big enough to properly train a CNN is still a problem [2]. The use of transfer learning by pre-trained CNN's can help avoid this problem, however the existing available pre-trained CNN's are trained with natural images with very different features from the texture-like mucosa patterns in the colonic polyp images.

In this paper, we explore the use of Convolutional Neural Networks (CNN's) pre-trained with natural images to use them as medical imaging feature extractors, specifically of rectal colon images for colonic polyps classification. Rather than directly train a CNN with medical images, we apply a simple transfer method using pre-trained Convolutional Neural Networks. The assumption is that the patterns learned in the original database can be used in colonoscopy images for colonic polyp classification. In particular, we explore 11 different architectures (from 5000 to 160 million parameters) and depths (different numbers of layers), describing and analyzing the effects of pre-trained CNN's in different acquisition modes of colonoscopy images (8 different databases). This study was motivated by recent studies in computer vision addressing the emerging technique of transfer learning using pre-trained CNN's presented in the next section.

2 CNN's in Medical Image Classification

In recent years there has been an increased interest in machine learning techniques that is based not on hand-engineered feature extractors but using raw data to learn the representations.

This type of model has been very successful in large annotated databases, such as ImageNet [16] dataset that contains around 1.2 million images divided into 1000 categories. For these tasks, it is common to have a large number of parameters (in order of millions), requiring a significant amount of processing power to train the Neural Network. The CNN's can learn through their numerous layers and millions of connections if they are trained with sufficient examples, which becomes a significant difficulty in the medical area [8]. This problem occurs because of the lack of large, annotated and publicly available medical image databases such as the existing natural image databases, so that is a difficult and costly task to acquire and annotate such images and due to the specific nature of different medical imaging modalities which seems to have different properties according to each modality [15].

Some current pattern recognition techniques set aside handcrafted feature extraction algorithms to feed a Deep Learning Neural Network directly with raw data simultaneously acting as features extractor and image classifier at the same time [8,23]. These networks use many consecutive convolutional layers followed by pooling layers that reduce the data dimensionality making it, concomitantly, invariant to geometric transformations. Such convolution filters (kernels) are built to act as feature extractors during the training process and recent research indicates that a satisfactorily trained CNN with a large database can perform properly when it is applied to other databases, which can mean that the kernels can turn into a universal feature extractor [23].

The works of Raza et al. [23] and Oquab et al. [20] suggest that the use of CNN's intermediate layer outputs can be used as input features to train other classifiers (such as support vector machines) for a number of other applications different from the original CNN obtaining a good performance. In fact, despite the difference between natural and medical images, some feature descriptors designed especially for natural images are used successfully in medical image detection and classification, for example: texture-based polyp detection [1], Fourier and Wavelet filters for colon classification [32], shape descriptors [14], local fractal dimension [13] for colonic polyp classification etc. In light of this, transfer learning that is a method used to harness the knowledge obtained by another task can be a good option to represent these kind of features.

Recently, works addressing the use of deep learning techniques in endoscopic images and videos are explored in many different ways, for example, to classify digestive organs in wireless capsule endoscopy images [34], detect lesions of endoscopy images [33] and automatically detect polyps in colonoscopy videos [22,27]. Also, pre-trained CNN's have been successfully used in the identification and pathology of X-ray and computer tomography modalities [8]. However, the application of transfer learning in endoscopic and colonoscopic images has not yet been exploited.

3   Materials and Methods

Using the inductive transfer learning, there are basically three types of strategies exploiting CNN's for medical image classification. Such strategies are described in the following and can be employed according to the intrinsic characteristics of each database [15].

When the available training database is large enough, diverse and very different from the database used in all the available pre-trained CNN's (in a case of transfer learning), the most appropriate approach would be to initialize the CNN weights randomly (training the **CNN from scratch**), and train it according to the medical image database for the kernels domain adaptation, that is, to find the best way to extract the features of the data in order to classify the images properly. This strategy, although ideal, is not widely used due to the lack of large and annotated medical image database publicly available for training the CNN.

Another alternative for large databases, but in this case, similar to a pre-trained CNN training database is the **CNN fine-tuning**. In fine-tuning the pre-trained network training continues with new entries (with a new database) for the weights to adjust properly to the new scenario reinforcing the more generic features with a lower probability of overfitting. This approach is also not widely applicable in case of medical image classification, again because of the limitation in the number of annotated medical images available for the appropriate network fine-tuning.

When the database is small, the best alternative is to use an **off-the-shelf CNN** [15]. In this case, using a pre-trained CNN, the last or next-to-last linear fully connected layer is removed and the remaining pre-trained CNN is used as a feature extractor to generate a feature vector for each input image from a different database. These feature vectors can be used to train a new classifier (such as an SVM) to classify the images correctly. If the original database is similar to the target database, the probability of the high-level features to describe the image correctly is high and relevant to this new database. If the target database is not so similar to the original, it can be more appropriate to use higher-level features, IE features from previous layers of CNN.

In this paper, we consider the knowledge transfer between natural images and medical images using off-the-shelf pre-trained CNN's. The CNN will project the target database samples into a vector space where the classes are more likely to be separable. This strategy was inspired by the work of Oquab et al. [20], which uses a pre-trained CNN in a large database (ImageNet) to classify images in a smaller database (Pascal VOC dataset) with improved results. Unlike that work, instead copy the weights of the original pre-trained CNN to the target CNN with additional layers, we use the pre-trained CNN to project data into a new feature space. This is done through the propagation of images from the colonic polyp database in the CNN, getting the resultant vector from the last CNN's layer and obtaining a new representation for each input sample. Subsequently, we use the feature vector set to train a linear classifier (for example support vector machines) in this representation to evaluate the results as used in [2,8].

To explore the use of different off-the-shelf CNN architectures for the computer-aided classification problem, we will describe below the elements to make the evaluation possible.

3.1   Data

The use of integrated endoscopic apparatus with high-resolution acquisition devices has been an important object of research in clinical decision support system area. With high-magnification colonoscopies is possible to acquire images up to 150-fold magnified, revealing the fine surface structure of the mucosa as well as small lesions. Recent work related to classification of colonic polyps used highly-detailed endoscopic images in combination with different technologies divided into three categories: high-definition endoscope (with or without staining the mucosa) combined with the i-Scan technology (1, 2, 3), high-magnification chromoendoscopy [9] and high-magnification endoscopy combined with narrow band imaging [7].

, Specifically, the i-Scan technology (Pentax) used in this work is an image processing technology consisting of the combination of surface enhancement and contrast enhancement aiming to help detect dysplastic areas and to accentuate mucosal surfaces [14].

There are three i-Scan modes available: i-Scan1, which includes surface enhancement and contrast enhancement, i-Scan2, that includes surface enhancement, contrast enhancement and tone enhancement and i-Scan3 that, besides including surface, contrast and tone enhancement, also increases lighting emphasizing the features of vascular visualization [32]. In this work we use an endoscopic image database (CC-i-Scan Database) with 8 different imaging modalities acquired by an HD endoscope (Pentax HiLINE HD+ 90i Colonoscope) with images of size 256×256 from video frames either using the i-Scan technology or without any computer virtual chromoendoscopy (¬CVC). Table 1 shows the number of images and patient per class in the different i-Scan modes. The mucosa is either stained or not stained. Despite the fact the frames being high-definition originally, the image size was chosen (i) to be large enough to describe a polyp and (ii) small enough to cover just one class of mucosa type (only healthy or only abnormal area). Also, the image labels (ground truth) were provided according to their histological diagnosis.

Table 1. Number of images and patients per class of the CC-i-Scan databases gathered with and without CC (staining) and computed virtual chromoendoscopy (CVC).

i-Scan mode	No staining				Staining			
	¬CVC	i-Scan1	i-Scan2	i-Scan3	¬CVC	i-Scan1	i-Scan2	i-Scan3
Non-neoplastic								
Number of images	39	25	20	31	42	53	32	31
Number of patients	21	18	15	15	26	31	23	19
Neoplastic								
Number of images	73	75	69	71	68	73	62	54
Number of patients	55	56	55	55	52	55	52	47
Total nr. of images	112	100	89	102	110	126	94	85

3.2　Pre-trained Convolutional Neural Networks Architectures

We mainly explore six different CNN architectures trained to perform classification in the ImageNet ILSVRC challenge data. The input of all tested pre-trained CNN's has size $224 \times 224 \times 3$ and the descriptions as well as the details of each CNN are given as follows:

- The **CNN VGG-VD** [25] uses a large number of layers with very small filters (3×3) divided into two architectures according to the number of their layers. The CNN **VGG-VD16** has 16 convolution layers and five pooling layers while the CNN **VGG-VD19** has 19 convolution layers, adding one more convolutional layer in three last sequences of convolutional layers. The fully connected layers have 4096 neurons followed by a softmax classifier with 1000 neurons corresponding to the number of classes in the ILSVRC classification. All the layers are followed by a rectifier linear unit (ReLU) layer to induce the sparsity in the hidden units and reduce the gradient vanishing problem.
- The **CNN-F** (also called Fast CNN) [4] is similar the CNN used by Krizhevsky et al. [16] with 5 convolutional layers. The input image size is 224×224 and

the fast processing is granted by the stride of 4 pixels in the first convolutional layer. The fully connected layers also have 4096 neurons as the CNN VGG-VD. Besides the original implementation, in this work we also used the MatConvnet implementation (beta17, [29]) of this architecture trained with batch normalization and minor differences in its default hyperparameters and called here **CNN-F MCN**.

- The **CNN-M** architecture (medium CNN) [4] also has 5 convolutional layers and 3 pooling layers. The number of filters is higher than the Fast CNN: 96 instead of 64 filters in the first convolution layer with a smaller size. We also use the MatConvNet implementation called **CNN-M MCN**.
- The **CNN-S** (slow CNN) [4] is related to the "accurate" network from the Overfeat package [24] and also has smaller filters with a stride of 2 pixels in the first convolutional layer. We also use the MatConvNet implementation called **CNN-S MCN**.
- The **AlexNet** CNN [16] has five convolutional layers, three pooling layers (after layer 2 and 5) and two fully connected layers. This architecture is similar to the CNN-F, however, with more filters in the convolutional layers. We also use the MatConvNet implementation called **AlexNet MCN**.
- The **GoogleLeNet** [26] CNN has the deepest and most complex architecture among all the other networks presented here. With two convolutional layers, two pooling layers and nine modules also called "inception" layers, this network was designed to avoid patch-alignment issues introducing more sparsity in the inception modules. Each module consists of six convolution layers and one pooling layer concatenating these filters of different sizes and dimensions into a single new filter.

3.3   Experimental Setup

In order to form the feature vector using the pre-trained CNNs, all images are scaled using bicubic interpolation to the required size for each network, in the case of this work: $224 \times 224 \times 3$. The vectors obtained from the linear layers of the CNN have size: 1024×1 for the GoogleLeNet CNN and 4096×1 for the other networks due to their architecture specificities.

To allow the CNN features comparison and evaluation, we compared them with the results obtained by some state-of-the-art feature extraction methods for the classification of colonic polyps [32] which are: Blob Shape adapted Gradient using Local Fractal Dimension method (**BSAG-LFD** [13]), Blob Shape and Contrast (**Blob SC** [14]), Discrete Shearlet Transform using the Weibull distribution (**Shearlet-Weibull** [5]), Gabor Wavelet Transform (**GWT Weibull** [32]), Local Color Vector Patterns (**LCVP** [11]) and Multi-Scale Block Local Binary Pattern (**MB-LBP** [11]). All these feature extraction methods (with the exception of BSAG-LFD) were applied to the three RGB channels to form the final feature vector space.

For the classical features, the classification accuracy is also computed using a SVM classifier however, with the original images (without resizing) trained using the Leave-One-Patient-out cross validation strategy as in [10] to make sure the classifier generalizes to unseen patients. This cross-validation is applied to the methods from the literature as well as to off-the-shelf CNN's features. The accuracy measure based on the percentage of images correctly classified in each class is used to allow an easy comparability of the results due to the high number of methods and databases to be compared.

4   Results and Discussion

The accuracy results for the colonic polyp classification in the 8 different databases are reported in Table 2. As can be seen, the results in Table 2 are divided into two groups: off-the-shelf features and concatenating them with state-of-the-art features.

Among the 11 pre-trained CNN investigated, the CNN that presents lower performance were GoogleLeNet, CNN-S and AlexNet MCN. These results may indicate that such networks themselves are not sufficient to be considered off-the-shelf feature extractors for the polyp classification task.

Table 2. Accuracies of the methods for the CC-i-Scan databases in %.

Methods	No staining				Staining				
	¬CVC	i-Scan1	i-Scan2	i-Scan3	¬CVC	i-Scan1	i-Scan2	i-Scan3	$\overline{X}$
1- CNN-F	86.16	89.33	80.65	88.41	86.52	81.40	84.22	80.62	84.66
2- CNN-M	87.45	90.67	81.38	83.58	87.99	89.55	87.40	90.53	87.31
3- CNN-S	88.03	90.00	87.01	77.33	87.25	82.68	87.40	75.54	84.41
4- CNN-F MCN	88.84	82.00	73.15	90.73	85.78	89.55	89.72	83.15	85.36
5- CNN-M MCN	89.53	90.67	88.88	94.66	86.97	89.29	87.40	90.53	**89.74**
6- CNN-S MCN	90.12	91.42	81.38	79.85	89.18	93.49	81.10	84.77	86.41
7- GoogleLeNet	79.65	90.67	72.43	74.51	88.27	80.46	75.60	84.08	80.70
8- VGG-VD16	87.45	85.33	86.38	79.65	92.47	89.80	95.26	92.38	88.59
9- VGG-VD19	83.49	82.67	83.88	87.71	92.47	83.98	94.46	85.59	86.78
10-AlexNet	91.40	87.33	75.65	89.32	87.71	83.03	84.22	79.24	84.73
11-AlexNet MCN	89.42	84.67	78.88	83.78	89.36	83.55	81.10	78.32	83.63
$\overline{X}$	87.41	87.70	80.88	84.50	88.54	86.07	86.17	84.06	85.67
13- Blob SC	77.67	83.33	82.10	75.22	59.28	78.83	66.13	59.83	72.79
14- Shearlet-Weibull	73.72	76.67	79.60	86.80	81.30	69.91	72.38	83.63	78.00
15- GWT-Weibull	79.75	78.67	70.25	84.28	81.30	74.54	77.17	83.39	78.66
16- LCVP	76.60	66.00	47.75	77.12	77.45	79.00	70.01	69.56	70.43
17- MB-LBP	78.26	80.67	81.38	83.37	69.29	70.60	77.22	78.32	77.38
$\overline{X}$	78.71	78.70	74.28	81.61	73.13	75.58	73.61	74.35	76.24
Concatenating 5/8	88.84	85.33	83.88	92.14	93.12	90.49	96.88	94.00	90.58
Concatenating 5/12	92.79	92.67	88.88	96.98	87.71	90.49	88.26	90.53	91.03
Concatenating 5/8/12	95.94	90.00	88.88	92.14	92.30	91.43	97.63	97.46	93.22
Concatenating 5/8/14	91.51	88.67	87.10	93.75	94.68	91.43	98.44	95.85	92.67
Concatenating 5/8/15	90.91	90.00	88.88	92.14	93.94	89.80	96.88	95.61	92.27
Concatenating 5/8/12/14	93.38	88.00	91.38	93.75	93.49	92.12	97.63	94.92	93.08
Concatenating 5/8/12/17	93.38	90.00	91.38	93.75	92.75	92.12	97.63	97.46	**93.55**

As it can be seen, the pre-trained CNN that presents the best result on average for the different imaging modalities ($\overline{X}$) is the CNN-M network trained with the MatConvNet parameters (89.74%) followed by the CNN VGG-VD16 (88.59%). These deep models with smaller filters generalize well with other datasets as it shown in [25], including texture recognition, which can explain the better results in the colonic polyp database. However, there is a high variability in the results and thus it is difficult to draw general conclusions.

Many results obtained by the pre-trained CNN's surpassed the classic feature extractors for colonic polyp classification in the literature. The database that presents the best results using off-the-shelf features is the database staining the mucosa without any i-Scan technology (88.54% on average). In the case of classical features, the database with the best result in the average is the database using the i-Scan3 technology without staining the mucosa (81.61%).

To investigate this difference in the results we asses the significance of them using the McNemar test [19]. By means of this test, we analyze if the images from a database are classified differently or similarly by the other methods. With a high accuracy it is suppose of that the methods will have a very similar response, so the significance level α must be small enough to differentiate between classifying an image as correct or incorrect.

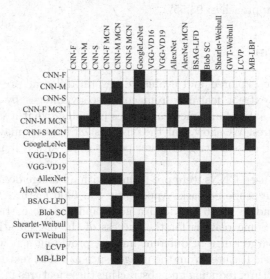

Fig. 2. Results of the McNemar test for the i-Scan3 database without staining. A black square in the matrix means that the methods are significantly different with significance level $\alpha = 0.01$. If the square is white then there is no significant difference between the methods.

The test is carried out on the database that presents the best results with the classic features (i-Scan3 without staining the mucosa) using significance level $\alpha = 0.01$. The results are presented in Fig. 2. It can be observed by the black squares that, among the pre-trained CNN's, the CNN-M MCN and GoogleLeNet present the most different results comparing to the other CNN's.

Also, in Fig. 2 when comparing the classical feature extraction methods with the CNN's features it can be seen that there is a quite different response among the results, especially for CNN-M MCN that is significantly different from all the classical methods with the exception of the Shearlet-Weilbull method.

The methods with high accuracy are not found to be significantly different which can indicate that, in these methods, almost the same images are classified wrong, independent of the extracted features.

Observing the features that are significantly different in Fig. 2 and with good results in Table 2 we decided to concatenate the feature vectors to see if the features can complement each other. It can be seen also in Table 2 that the two most successful CNN's (CNN-M MCN and VGG-VD16) are significantly different from each other and, at the same time, the CNN-M MCN is significantly different to BSAG-LFD features which, among the classical results, presents the best results.

Based on this difference, the three feature vectors (CNN-M, CNN-M MCN and BSAG-LFD) were concatenated and the results presents a high accuracy on average: 93.22%. When we add to the vector one more classical feature (MB-LBP) that is also significantly different to CNN-M MCN, the result outperforms all the previous approaches: 93.55%.

5   Conclusion

In this paper, we explored and evaluated several different pre-trained CNN's architectures to extract features from colonoscopy images by the knowledge transfer between natural and medical images providing what it is called off-the-shelf CNNs features. We show that the off-the shelf features may be well suited for the automatic classification of colon polyps even with a limited amount of data.

The different used CNNs were pre-trained with an image domain completely different from the proposed task. Apparently the 4096 features extracted from CNN-M MCN and VGG-16 provided a good and generic extractor of colonic polyps features. Some reasons for the success of the classification include the training with a large range of different images, providing a powerful extractor joining the intrinsic features from the images such as color, texture and shape in the same architecture, reducing and abstracting these features in just one vector.

Also, the combination of classical features with off-the-shelf features yields good prediction results complementing each other. We believe that this strategy could be used in other endoscopic databases such as automatic classification of celiac disease. Besides that, this approach will be explored in future work to also detect polyps in video frames and the performance in real time applications will be evaluated. It can be concluded that Deep Learning through Convolutional Neural Networks is becoming essentially the most favorite candidate in almost all pattern recognition tasks.

References

1. Ameling, S., Wirth, S., Paulus, D., Lacey, G., Vilarino, F.: Texture-based polyp detection in colonoscopy. In: Meinzer, H.-P., Deserno, T.M., Handels, H., Tolxdorff, T. (eds.) Bildverarbeitung für die Medizin 2009. Informatik aktuell, pp. 346–350. Springer, Heidelberg (2009)
2. Bar, Y., Diamant, I., Wolf, L., Lieberman, S., Konen, E., Greenspan, H.: Chest pathology detection using deep learning with non-medical training. In: 2015 IEEE 12th International Symposium on Biomedical Imaging (ISBI), pp. 294–297, April 2015
3. Bernal, J., Schez, J., Vilario, F.: Towards automatic polyp detection with a polyp appearance model. Pattern Recognit. **45**(9), 3166–3182 (2012). Best Papers of Iberian Conference on Pattern Recognition and Image Analysis (IbPRIA 2011)
4. Chatfield, K., Simonyan, K., Vedaldi, A., Zisserman, A.: Return of the devil in the details: delving deep into convolutional nets. In: British Machine Vision Conference, BMVC 2014, Nottingham, 1–5 September 2014
5. Dong, Y., Tao, D., Li, X., Ma, J., Pu, J.: Texture classification and retrieval using shearlets and linear regression. IEEE Trans. Cybern. **45**(3), 358–369 (2015)
6. Ribeiro E., Uhl, A., Häfner, M.: Colonic polyp classification with convolutional neural networks. In: 2016 29th International Symposium on Computer-Based Medical Systems (CBMS), June 2016
7. Ganz, M., Yang, X., Slabaugh, G.: Automatic segmentation of polyps in colonoscopic narrow-band imaging data. IEEE Trans. Biomed. Eng. **59**(8), 2144–2151 (2012)
8. Ginneken, B., Setio, A., Jacobs, C., Ciompi, F.: Off-the-shelf convolutional neural network features for pulmonary nodule detection in computed tomography scans. In: 12th IEEE International Symposium on Biomedical Imaging, ISBI 2015, Brooklyn, 16–19 April 2015, pp. 286–289 (2015)
9. Häfner, M., Kwitt, R., Uhl, A., Gangl, A., Wrba, F., Vécsei, A.: Feature extraction from multi-directional multi-resolution image transformations for the classification of zoom-endoscopy images. Pattern Anal. Appl. **12**(4), 407–413 (2009)
10. Häfner, M., Liedlgruber, M., Maimone, S., Uhl, A., Vécsei, A., Wrba, F.: Evaluation of cross-validation protocols for the classification of endoscopic images of colonic polyps. In: 2012 25th International Symposium on Computer-Based Medical Systems (CBMS), pp. 1–6, June 2012
11. Häfner, M., Liedlgruber, M., Uhl, A., Vécsei, A., Wrba, F.: Color treatment in endoscopic image classification using multi-scale local color vector patterns. Med. Image Anal. **16**(1), 75–86 (2012)
12. Häfner, M., Liedlgruber, M., Uhl, A., Vécsei, A., Wrba, F.: Delaunay triangulation-based pit density estimation for the classification of polyps in high-magnification chromo-colonoscopy. Comput. Methods Programs Biomed. **107**(3), 565–581 (2012)
13. Häfner, M., Tamaki, T., Tanaka, S., Uhl, A., Wimmer, G., Yoshida, S.: Local fractal dimension based approaches for colonic polyp classification. Med. Image Anal. **26**(1), 92–107 (2015)
14. Häfner, M., Uhl, A., Wimmer, G.: A novel shape feature descriptor for the classification of polyps in HD colonoscopy. In: Menze, B., Langs, G., Montillo, A., Kelm, M., Müller, H., Tu, Z. (eds.) MCV 2013. LNCS, vol. 8331, pp. 205–213. Springer, Heidelberg (2014). doi:10.1007/978-3-319-05530-5_20

15. Shin, H., Roth, H., Gao, M., Lu, L., Xu, Z., Nogues, I., Yao, J., Mollura, D., Summers, R.: Deep convolutional neural networks for computer-aided detection: CNN architectures, dataset characteristics and transfer learning. CoRR, abs/1602.03409 (2016)
16. Alex K., Sutskever, I., Hinton, G.E.: Imagenet classification with deep convolutional neural networks. In: Advances in Neural Information Processing Systems, vol. 25, pp. 1097–1105. Curran Associates Inc. (2012)
17. Kato, S., Fu, K.I., Sano, Y., Fujii, T., Saito, Y., Matsuda, T., Koba, I., Yoshida, S., Fujimori, T.: Magnifying colonoscopy as a non-biopsy technique for differential diagnosis of non-neoplastic and neoplastic lesions. World J. Gastroenterol. 12(9), 1416–1420 (2006)
18. Kudo, S., Hirota, S., Nakajima, T.: Colorectal tumours and pit pattern. J. Clin. Pathol. 10, 880–885 (1994)
19. McNemar, Q.: Note on the sampling error of the difference between correlated proportions or percentages. Psychometrika 12(2), 153–157 (1947)
20. Oquab, M., Bottou, L., Laptev, I., Sivic, J.: Learning and transferring mid-level image representations using convolutional neural networks. In: 2014 IEEE Conference on Computer Vision and Pattern Recognition, CVPR 2014, Columbus, 23–28 June 2014, pp. 1717–1724 (2014)
21. Sun, Y.P., Sargent, D., Spofford, I., Vosburgh, K.G., A-Rahim, Y.: A colon video analysis framework for polyp detection. IEEE Trans. Biomed. Eng. 59(5), 1408–1418 (2012)
22. Park, S.Y., Sargent, D.: Colonoscopic polyp detection using convolutional neural networks. In: Proceedings of SPIE, vol. 9785, p. 978528 (2016)
23. Razavian, A., Azizpour, H., Sullivan, J., Carlsson, S.: CNN features off-the-shelf: an astounding baseline for recognition. In: IEEE Conference on Computer Vision and Pattern Recognition, CVPR Workshops 2014, Columbus, 23–28 June 2014, pp. 512–519 (2014)
24. Sermanet, P., Eigen, D., Zhang, X., Mathieu, M., Fergus, R., LeCun, Y.: Overfeat: integrated recognition, localization and detection using convolutional networks. CoRR, abs/1312.6229 (2013)
25. Simonyan, K., Zisserman, A.: Very deep convolutional networks for large-scale image recognition. CoRR, abs/1409.1556 (2014)
26. Szegedy, C., Liu, W., Jia, Y., Sermanet, P., Reed, S., Anguelov, D., Erhan, D., Vanhoucke, V., Rabinovich, A.: Going deeper with convolutions. In: Computer Vision and Pattern Recognition (CVPR) (2015)
27. Tajbakhsh, N., Gurudu, S.R., Liang, J.: Automatic polyp detection in colonoscopy videos using an ensemble of convolutional neural networks. In: 2015 IEEE 12th International Symposium on Biomedical Imaging (ISBI), pp. 79–83, April 2015
28. Tajbakhsh, N., Gurudu, S.R., Liang, J.: Automated polyp detection in colonoscopy videos using shape and context information. IEEE Trans. Med. Imaging 35(2), 630–644 (2016)
29. Vedaldi, A., Lenc, K.: Matconvnet - convolutional neural networks for MATLAB. CoRR, abs/1412.4564 (2014)
30. Yi, W., Tavanapong, W., Wong, J., Oh, J., de Groen, P.C.: Part-based multi-derivative edge cross-sectional profiles for polyp detection in colonoscopy. IEEE J. Biomed. Health Inform. 18(4), 1379–1389 (2014)
31. Wang, Y., Tavanapong, W., Wong, J., Oh, J.H., de Groen, P.C.: Polyp-alert: near real-time feedback during colonoscopy. Comput. Methods Programs Biomed. 120(3), 164–179 (2015)

32. Wimmer, G., Tamaki, T., Tischendorf, J.J.W., Häfner, M., Yoshida, S., Tanaka, S., Uhl, A.: Directional wavelet based features for colonic polyp classification. Med. Image Anal. **31**, 16–36 (2016)
33. Zhu, R., Zhang, R., Xue, D.: Lesion detection of endoscopy images based on convolutional neural network features. In: 2015 8th International Congress on Image and Signal Processing (CISP), pp. 372–376, October 2015
34. Zou, Y., Li, L., Wang, Y., Yu, J., Li, Y., Deng, W.J.: Classifying digestive organs in wireless capsule endoscopy images based on deep convolutional neural network. In: 2015 IEEE International Conference on Digital Signal Processing (DSP), pp. 1274–1278, July 2015

Probe Tracking and Its Application in Automatic Acquisition Using a Trans-Esophageal Ultrasound Robot

Shuangyi Wang[1]([⊠]), Davinder Singh[2], David Lau[1], Kiran Reddy[1], Kaspar Althoefer[3], Kawal Rhode[1], and Richard J. Housden[1]

[1] Division of Imaging Science and Biomedical Engineering,
King's College London, London, UK
shuangyi.wang@kcl.ac.uk
[2] Xtronics Ltd., Gravesend, UK
[3] Department of Informatics, King's College London, London, UK

Abstract. Robotic trans-esophageal echocardiography (TEE) has many advantages over the traditional manual control approach during cardiac surgical procedures in terms of stability, remote operation, and radiation safety. To further improve the usability of the robotic approach, development of an intelligent system using automatic acquisition of ultrasound images is proposed. This is addressed using a view planning platform in which the robot is controlled according to a pre-planned path during the acquisition. Considering the real mechanical movement, feedback of the probe position is essential in ensuring the success of the automatic acquisition. In this paper, we present a tracking method using the combination of an electromagnetic (EM) tracking system and image-based registration for the purpose of feedback control used in the automatic acquisition. Phantom experiments were performed to evaluate the accuracy and reliability of the tracking and the automatic acquisition. The results indicate a reliable performance of the tracking method. As for automatic acquisition, the mean positioning error in the near field of ultrasound where most structures of clinical interest are located is 10.44 mm. This phantom study is encouraging for the eventual clinical application of robotic-based automatic TEE acquisition.

1 Introduction

Trans-esophageal ultrasound is a manually controlled imaging modality widely used for diagnosing heart disease and guiding cardiac surgical procedures [1]. The on-site operation of the probe usually requires operators standing for long periods of time and wearing heavy radiation-protection shielding when X-ray is utilized during the surgery [2]. Apart from the inconvenience and tedium of the manual control, the need for highly specialized skills is always a barrier for reliable and repeatable acquisition of ultrasound. Accordingly, there is a need for an automatic TEE system and method to acquire the desired imaging based on the user's request. Though numerous works have been presented for robotic ultrasound as reviewed in [3], there is no solution for automatic heart scanning

© Springer International Publishing AG 2017
T. Peters et al. (Eds.): CARE 2016, LNCS 10170, pp. 14–23, 2017.
DOI: 10.1007/978-3-319-54057-3_2

with TEE produced so far due to the complexity of heart imaging and the unavailability of a robot specifically designed for this task.

A recently developed robotic system for TEE has made remote control possible [4] and we have subsequently proposed an automatic acquisition workflow (as shown in Fig. 1) [5] using this robot based on a view-planning platform for path-panning and an ultrasound-to-MR registration method [6] for locating the probe position when applying feedback. However, in the workflow described in [5], the probe tracking method based on registering 3-D echo images to pre-scanned MR models requires a close estimate of the probe pose. This was estimated based on the robotic kinematics, which could result in failures because the mechanical performance of the probe driven by the robot mechanism within the real esophagus could be different to the kinematics in the simulation environment. Therefore, a method of more reliable tracking of the probe is a key component for automatic acquisition to be clinically transferable. As an alternative option, EM tracking systems are widely used for medical device tracking and have been reported for tracking the TEE probe [7]. However, registering the EM tracking coordinates to the patient coordinates is required which is difficult to achieve using the EM tracking system on its own and the accuracy of EM tracking could also be influenced by the electromagnetic environment.

To solve the problem of reliable tracking, we introduce a method to combine the EM tracking system with image-based registration for probe tracking and integrate this method into the workflow as shown in Fig. 1. This tracking method is tested with a phantom experiment in which the tracking information provides feedback for the robot. The performances of the combined tracking method and the automatic acquisition are analyzed and discussed. In this paper, the robotic system and the view-based motion planning are briefly reviewed in Sect. 2.1. Details of the new probe tracking method are presented in Sect. 2.2. The utilization of this new tracking method in feedback position control, relying on the inverse kinematics, is introduced in Sect. 2.3. Based on these methods, experiments, results, discussion and conclusions are presented in the subsequent sections.

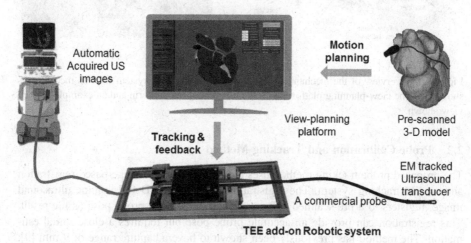

Fig. 1. Overview of the TEE add-on robotic system and the automatic acquisition workflow.

2 Materials and Methods

2.1 Robotic System and View-Based Motion Planning

An overview of the robotic system is shown in Fig. 2(a). The add-on TEE robot holds the probe handle and manipulates four degrees of freedom (DOFs) that are available in manual handling of the probe, including the rotation about and translation along the length of the TEE probe and additional manipulators with 2-DOFs to steer the probe head. The remote operation of the probe is via Bluetooth communication. More details of the design of the robotic system can be found in [4].

In the view-planning platform (Fig. 2(b)) described in [5], an automatically seg-mented heart 3-D model from the pre-scanned MR image, the corresponding manually segmented esophagus center line, and the virtual model of the TEE probe head can be loaded and viewed intuitively. The forward kinematics of the probe is modeled and the corresponding virtual 2-D ultrasound images are displayed based on the given robotic parameters [4]. By defining targeted views based on the virtual ultrasound image outputs, sets of robotic parameters, along with planed paths for the robotic movements, can be obtained.

In addition, the view-planning platform has the capability of auto-patient adaption, in which case standard TEE views of patient-specific data can be automatically obtained based on registration and optimization methods. This function allows rapid motion planning of the acquisition if standard TEE views in the protocol are required as targets. Details of the auto-patient adaption method can be found in [5].

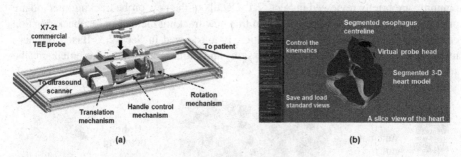

Fig. 2. (a) Overview of the mechanical design of the robotic TEE system with its mechanisms shown. (b) The view-planning platform with the function of the platform and an example defined view shown.

2.2 Probe Calibration and Tracking Method

The proposed probe tracking method uses the combination of image-based registration and an EM tracking system. The registration [6] takes a 3-D full-volume ultrasound image, registers to a pre-scanned MR image and obtains the probe pose as the result. This registration can provide an accurate probe pose but requires a close initial esti-mation. The method has previously been shown to have a capture range of 9 mm [9].

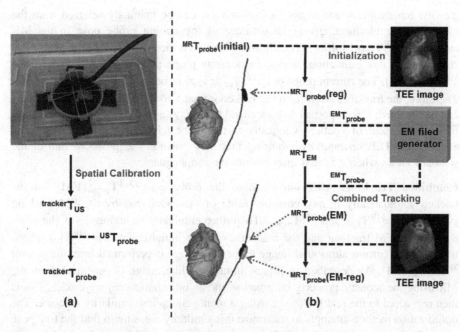

Fig. 3. (a) Experimental setup and workflow for the calibration of the probe. (b) Flow diagram of the tracking method used in the TEE automatic acquisition.

We therefore introduce EM tracking to the workflow, which typical has accuracy within this range, to provide the initial estimation and ensure the success of the registration.

Spatial Calibration. In the workflow, EM tracking is done using the Aurora Electromagnetic Measurement System (Northern Digital Inc, Waterloo, Canada). An EM sensor has been mounted onto the tip of the probe. Spatial calibration of the ultrasound image to the EM tracker was by a simple registration-based method using a phantom comprising several crossed wires [8]. The experimental setup and workflow for the calibration are shown in Fig. 3(a). 3-D images of the wires were acquired at different positions and orientations, and the straight lines and crossing points of the wires were extracted manually. The calibration transformation $^{\mathrm{tracker}}T_{\mathrm{US}}$ was then solved for iteratively to minimise the misalignment of the extracted wires in each position. From this the targeted transformation $^{\mathrm{tracker}}T_{\mathrm{probe}}$ was obtained using a prior known transformation from the probe coordinates to the ultrasound image coordinates. Using this spatial calibration, a measured pose of the EM tracker in the EM coordinates (defined by the Aurora field generator) can be converted to the pose of the probe in the EM coordinates $^{\mathrm{EM}}T_{\mathrm{probe}}$.

Initialization. In order to provide the probe pose in the MR coordinates, another calibration between the EM coordinates and the MR coordinates must be obtained. This can be done at the time when the probe is manually inserted into the esophagus at a random starting pose with the probe pointing towards the heart. By visually looking at the first output ultrasound image, a similar view can be manually selected from the view-planning platform, giving an estimate of the current probe pose in the MR coordinates $^{MR}T_{probe}(\text{initial})$. The ultrasound image is then registered to the MR image starting from this estimation, giving an accurate probe pose in the MR coordinates $^{MR}T_{probe}(\text{reg})$. The current probe pose $^{EM}T_{probe}$ is also measured from the EM system. Therefore, the transformation from the EM coordinates to the MR coordinates $^{MR}T_{EM}$ can be obtained. It is important to understand that this is a once-only manual operation for each TEE scan of a patient. Clinically, this could be achieved relatively easily by an experienced TEE operator by requiring that they position the probe to one of the standard views when it is first inserted into the esophagus.

Combined Tracking. After initialization, the probe pose $^{MR}T_{probe}(\mathbf{EM})$ can be tracked automatically in any position inside of the esophagus by the EM tracking system using $^{MR}T_{EM}$ and $^{EM}T_{probe}$. To further eliminate the influence of the environment on EM tracking and the inaccuracy of the initial calibration $^{MR}T_{EM}$, registration of the current ultrasound image to the MR image is performed from the current $^{MR}T_{probe}(\mathbf{EM})$. As described in [6], an ultrasound-like image is generated from the MR using the acoustic property information and an ultrasound imaging model. This is then registered to the real US image using a monogenic phase similarity measure. The optimization method attempts to maximize this similarity measure to find the true pose of the TEE probe relative to the MR coordinates $^{MR}T_{probe}(\mathbf{EM} - \mathbf{reg})$, which is used to provide feedback for the robot control. The overview of the initialization and combined tracking are shown in Fig. 3(b).

2.3   Inverse Kinematics and Feedback

The tracking result is used as feedback information for the robotic system to adjust the parameters required to obtain the targeted positions. In order to find the robotic parameters' offsets between the current pose and the targeted pose, an inverse kinematic model is proposed using a gradient decent search strategy based on the forward kinematics reported before. The search strategy defines a single objective function in order to optimize the robotic parameters $p = (x, \theta, \alpha, \beta)$, where x is the translation parameter, θ is the axial rotation parameter, and α, β are the bi-directional bending parameters. The forward kinematics, denoted as F, gives the transformation from the probe coordinates to the MR coordinates:

$$^{MR}T_{probe} = F(\mathbf{p}) = F(x, \theta, \alpha, \beta) \tag{1}$$

Detailed information on the forward kinematics is given in [4]. The objective function uses the four corners of the probe transducer face as reference points, denoted as $\mathbf{R_i}$. The current pose of the probe is denoted as $^{MR}T_{probe^*}$, and the objective function $f(\mathbf{p})$ used for optimization is defined as follows:

$$f(\mathbf{p}) = -\frac{1}{4}\sum_{i=1}^{4}\left\|{}^{MR}T_{probe}{}^{*}R_i - F(\mathbf{p})R_i\right\| \tag{2}$$

During the search and step approach, the parameter p_i in the parameter space $\mathbf{p}$ which gives the maximum partial derivative will be selected as the step parameter to be updated. The best step direction $d_i = -\nabla f(p_i)/\|\nabla f(p_i)\|$ in the step direction space $\mathbf{d}$ is the forward direction of the selected parameter. The step size, σ, is initially defined based on the dimension scale of each parameter and then reduced after each convergence when $\nabla f(p_i) = 0$. A new parameter set $\mathbf{p}_+$ is of the form:

$$\mathbf{p}_+ = \mathbf{p} + \sigma \cdot \mathbf{d} \tag{3}$$

The search strategy starts from $\mathbf{p} = \mathbf{0}$ and ends when $f(\mathbf{p})$ reaches its minimum preset value. The final parameter set $\mathbf{p}^*$, representing the current pose of the probe, is the output of the inverse kinematics. With the tracking information and the inverse kinematics, a simple feedback position controller is designed as shown in Fig. 4. Based on the result from the previous work [5], the cycle of measurement and adjustment is executed only one time, which has been shown to effectively improve the accuracy.

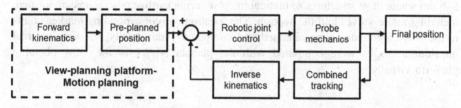

Fig. 4. Feedback position controller based on the tracking and kinematics of the TEE robot.

2.4 Automatic Acquisition Experiment

A phantom experiment was designed to test the proposed tracking method and its performance in automatic TEE acquisition. A custom phantom was built in order to provide a simulation environment for the TEE approach. This phantom includes a silicone tube representing the esophagus and a commercial ultrasound/MRI heart phantom (Computerized Imaging Reference Systems, Incorporated (CIRS), USA.) used for imaging. The heart and silicone tube model of the phantom were extracted from the pre-scanned MR image and loaded into the view-based robot planning platform. Based on featured structures (chambers, valves, vessels) shown in either long-axis view or short-axis view, five views were defined and the corresponding probe poses and robotic parameters were recorded. Mechanically, a special link mechanism was designed in order to lead the endoscopic portion of the TEE probe translating into the phantom. The experimental setup is show in Fig. 5.

During the experiment, the initial calibration between the EM coordinates and the MR coordinates was performed at the very beginning using the method described in

Sect. 2.2. After initialization, the probe was tracked by the proposed tracking method. Based on the pre-planned poses of the probe, the robotic system was actuated, driving the probe towards the targeted poses. When the probe arrived, the tracked probe pose was used as feedback information with the inverse kinematics method described in Sect. 2.3. The adjustments of the probe parameters were calculated and performed, and the ultrasound image recorded. The experiment was repeated three times with different random initial poses of the probe.

For post-processing, to understand the improvement in accuracy using the combined tracking method over the EM tracking method, the tracked probe poses reported by the EM tracking system $^{MR}T_{probe}(EM)$ and the combined tracking method $^{MR}T_{probe}(EM - reg)$ were compared. Root sum square (RSS) of the differences between the X-, Y-, and Z-axes rotation and translation components were calculated after decomposing each matrix. To understand the need for using the EM tracking system to provide the initial estimate of registration for tracking, we used robot kinematics as an alternative initialization for the registrations and compared the success rate with the proposed combined tracking method. The accuracy of automatic acquisition was quantified by comparing the final probe pose determined by registration $^{MR}T_{probe}(EM - reg)$ with the planned probe pose $^{MR}T_{probe}(\mathbf{planned})$. 60 marker points were defined in the ultrasound image field of view ($90° * 90°$ cone) at a depth of 5–6 cm where most structures of clinical interest during cardiac procedures are located, including major valves and the septum. The locations of corresponding marker points in the MR coordinates were obtained and compared. Additionally, the acquired real ultrasound images were compared with the planned views in the view planning platform visually.

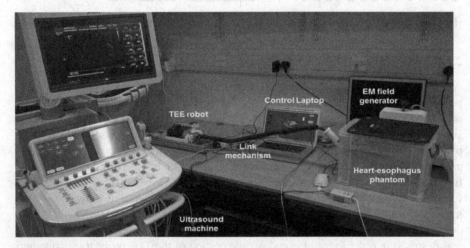

Fig. 5. Experimental setup for the automatic acquisition using the TEE robot, custom heart-esophagus phantom, and the EM tracking system.

3 Results

Results from the experiments indicate that the proposed tracking method is suitable for the robotic-based automatic TEE acquisition. Figure 6(a) shows one of the tracking examples where the EM tracking provided a close estimation and the image-based registration calculated an accurate probe pose. Visual examination of the registration results found that the combined registration result could not be improved by manual adjustments, whereas the EM-only registration had some clear misalignment. Quantitatively, the proposed combined tracking method has a relatively high tracking accuracy with a median registration error of 2.9 mm. This has been shown previously from the investigation of the registration method itself in [9]. Therefore, the combined tracking result is used as the reference to compare with the EM tracking result. The error in the EM tracking method compared to the combined result indicates an

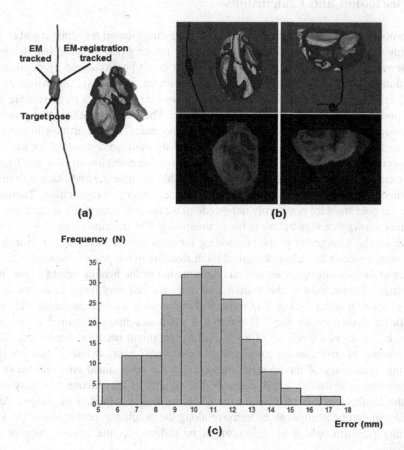

Fig. 6. (a) Example of tracking with target probe pose (black), EM tracked pose (green), and EM-registration tracked pose (white) shown. (b) Examples of automatic acquisition results with planned view (top row) and acquired real ultrasound images (bottom row) shown. (c) Histogram of the error at 5–6 cm depth. (Color figure online)

improvement of 7.96 mm and 3.41° in tracking accuracy. The success rate is 11 out of 15 (73%) using the kinematics to provide the initial estimate of registration while all registrations succeed (100%) using the EM tracking result as the initial estimate of registration. For the performance of the automatic acquisition, the ultrasound image was overlaid on the MR segmentation data in order to intuitively compare the acquired ultrasound views with the views originally defined in the view planning software (example views are shown in Fig. 6(b)). The results show that all planned structures were in the 3-D field of view and most of the center slices of the obtained ultrasound images align with the original slice planned in the view planning platform. Quantitatively, the overall error of marker points defined in the ultrasound field of view at the depth of interest over all three experiments is 10.44 ± 2.30 mm (mean ± standard deviation). A histogram of this error is shown in Fig. 6(c).

4 Discussion and Conclusions

The proposed combined tracking method using the image-based registration and an EM tracking system together enables a more accurate tracking performance than using the EM sensor alone. This is because the EM sensor could be influenced by the metallic environment and an inaccurate calibration. Compared with using kinematics as the initial estimate of registration, the EM tracking system provides a more reliable estimate and ensures the success rate of the tracking. Therefore we believe the proposed combined tracking method is suitable for the automatic TEE acquisition in terms of both accuracy and reliability. It should be noted that our gold standard for the error measurement of the tracking method was to run the registration from a good initial alignment, and then to manually correct any visible alignment errors, although in the experiment there was almost no visible misalignment after this registration. Therefore, while the gold standard is not truly independent, we are confident that it is accurate, and certainly shows that registration is better than using EM tracking alone.

As for the accuracy of probe positioning for automatic acquisition, the error in the ultrasound space at the depth of clinical interested due to the probe positioning error is similar to the amount of movement and deformation of the beating heart (1 cm). With this range of error, most of the desired anatomies are still very likely to remain in the field of view in either 2-D or 3-D mode. However, such a deviation might still cause significant challenges for the 2-D mode if a small structure is required in the view plane. In that case, a precision of a few millimeters might need to be achieved. There are a number of error sources contributing to the overall error, including the error from tracking, inaccuracy of the inverse kinematics in the constrained environment of the silicone tube, and mechanical movement. The rigidity of the silicone tube may mean that the feedback is less effective in the phantom than in a human esophagus. Additionally, the probe is constrained to move along the esophagus center line in the view planning platform, which in reality might be different in the silicone tube or real esophagus.

In this paper, we have proposed a method of probe tracking using an EM tracking system and image-based registration to work with a TEE robot. This method is particularly developed for the application of automatic TEE acquisition. Results from the experiment demonstrated the feasibility of the tracking method and proved the new concept of automatic TEE acquisition in a phantom. To further evaluate the method in the human body, specially preserved cadavers using the Thiel embalming method [10] will be employed and the whole workflow will be evaluated in a more realistic clinical scenario. The accuracy requirements for the automatic TEE acquisition workflow in this less rigid environment can be re-evaluated based on a qualitative study judging whether the planned structures are successfully obtained in a real human body. In addition, further developments in automation, particularly in the initialization, will be necessary for clinical translation of the workflow.

Acknowledgements. This work was funded by the KCL NIHR Healthcare Technology Centre and KCL-China Scholarship Scheme. This research was also supported by the National Institute for Health Research (NIHR) Biomedical Research Centre at Guy's and St. Thomas' NHS Foundation Trust and King's College London. The views expressed are those of the authors and not necessarily those of the NHS, the NIHR or the Department of Health.

References

1. Vegas, A., Meineri, M.: Three-dimensional transesophageal echocardiography is a major advance for intraoperative clinical management of patients undergoing cardiac surgery, a core review. Anesth. Analg. **110**, 1548–1573 (2010)
2. Goldstein, J.A., Balter, S., Cowley, M., Hodgson, J., Klein, L.W.: Occupational hazards of interventional cardiologists: prevalence of orthopedic health problems in contemporary practice. Cathet. Cardiovasc. Interv. **63**, 407–411 (2004)
3. Priester, A., Natarajan, S., Culjat, M.: Robotic ultrasound systems in medicine. IEEE Trans. Ultrason. Ferroelectr. Freq. Contr. **60**, 507–523 (2013)
4. Wang, S., Housden, J., Singh, D., Althoefer, K., Rhode, K.: Design, testing and modelling of a novel robotic system for trans-oesophageal ultrasound. Int. J. Med. Robot. Comput. Assist. Surg. **12**(3), 342–354 (2015)
5. Wang, S., Singh, D., Johnson, D., Althoefer, K., Rhode, K., Housden, J.: Robotic ultrasound: view planning, tracking, and automatic acquisition of trans-esophageal echocardiography. IEEE Robot. Autom. Magaz. **23**(4), 118–127 (2016)
6. King, A.P., Rhode, K.S., Ma, Y., Yao, C., Jansen, C., Razavi, R., Penney, G.P.: Registering preprocedure volumetric images with intraprocedure 3-D ultrasound using an ultrasound imaging model. IEEE Trans. Med. Imaging **29**, 924–937 (2010)
7. Lang, A., Jain, A., Parthasarathy, V.: Calibration of EM sensors for spatial tracking of 3D ultrasound probes. INTECH Open Access Publisher (2012)
8. Bergmeir, C., Seitel, M., Frank, C., Simone, R.D., Meinzer, H.-P., Wolf, I.: Comparing calibration approaches for 3D ultrasound probes. Int. J. Comput. Assist. Radiol. Surg. **4**, 203–213 (2008)
9. Housden, R.J., et al.: Three-modality registration for guidance of minimally invasive cardiac interventions. In: Ourselin, S., Rueckert, D., Smith, N. (eds.) FIMH 2013. LNCS, vol. 7945, pp. 158–165. Springer, Heidelberg (2013). doi:10.1007/978-3-642-38899-6_19
10. Healy, S.E., Rai, B.P., Biyani, C.S., Eisma, R., Soames, R.W., Nabi, G.: Thiel embalming method for cadaver preservation: a review of new training model for urologic skills training. Urology **85**, 499–504 (2015)

Hybrid Tracking and Matching Algorithm for Mosaicking Multiple Surgical Views

Chisato Takada[1($\boxtimes$)], Toshiyuki Suzuki[2], Ahmed Afifi[3], and Toshiya Nakaguchi[4]

[1] School of Engineering, Chiba University, Chiba, Japan
takadachisato@chiba-u.jp
[2] Graduate School of Engineering, Chiba University, Chiba, Japan
[3] Faculty of Computers and Information, Menoufia University, Shebin El-kom, Menoufia, Egypt
[4] Research Center for Frontier Medical Engineering, Chiba University, Chiba, Japan

Abstract. In recent years, laparoscopic surgery has become major surgery due to several advantages for patients. However, it has disadvantages for operators because of the narrow surgical field of view. To solve this problem, our group proposed camera-retractable trocar which can obtain multiple surgical viewpoints while maintaining the minimally invasiveness. The purpose of this study is to obtain a wide visual panoramic view by utilizing image mosaicking of camera-retractable trocar viewpoints videos. We utilize feature points tracking in different videos to generate panoramic video independent of inter-cameras overlap and to increase mosaicking speed and robustness. We evaluate tracking accuracy according to several conditions and mosaicking accuracy according to overlap size. In contrast to the conventional mosaicking approach, the proposed approach can produce panoramic image even in the case of 0% inter-cameras overlap. Additionally, the proposed approach is fast enough for clinical use.

1 Introduction

Laparoscopic surgery, one of the minimally invasive surgeries (MIS), has several advantages for patients. For example, patients would feel less postoperative pain because of the small surgical wound, can early discharge and can early return to their social activities. However, this surgery has disadvantages for operators because of the narrow surgical field of view. Also, the safety improvement of this surgery is strongly required owing to concern for the medical accidents occurred in recent years. As one of the countermeasures for this problem, it has been demanded to realize a wide visual field such as abdominal surgery maintaining the minimally invasiveness that is an advantage of laparoscopic surgery. In the case of endoscopic surgery or robotic assisted surgery, image mosaicking and image mapping are proposed to achieve a wide visual field [1, 2].

In the present laparoscopic surgery, operators insert a laparoscope into a port and display a single viewpoint video on a monitor. It is a major operative procedure. In recent years, several mosaicking methods are proposed to expand the surgical view. These methods usually use monocular tracking [3–6], or stereo imaging devices [7]. However, these methods extend the field of view using static panorama images and do not provide a real extended view of the operation site. To achieve a real wider visual field, we must

© Springer International Publishing AG 2017
T. Peters et al. (Eds.): CARE 2016, LNCS 10170, pp. 24–35, 2017.
DOI: 10.1007/978-3-319-54057-3_3

observe intraperitoneal conditions from new ports other than the laparoscope port. Camera-retractable trocar is proposed by Okubo et al. [8] to invasively provide multiple surgical views. Trocar is a surgical instrument that is inserted through abdominal wall to secure forceps ports and to keep abdominal air pressure. Camera-retractable trocar, shown in Fig. 1(a), (b), has a miniature camera which can be retracted or expanded at the end of the trocar. It is possible to obtain several videos of different viewpoints from the camera-retractable trocar. Therefore, it is possible to obtain multiple surgical viewpoints videos while maintaining the minimally invasiveness which is an advantage of laparoscopic surgery. Although these advantage of camera-retractable trocar, observing multiple views at the same time may cause confusion specially in the case of overlapped views.

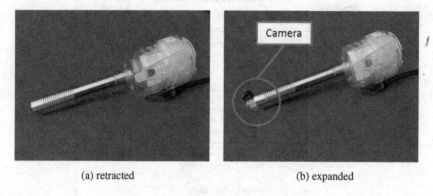

(a) retracted   (b) expanded

Fig. 1. Camera-retractable trocar.

In this study, therefore, we tend to utilize camera-retractable trocar views to provide a more realistic expanded surgical view. Supposing the situation that two camera-retractable trocars are placed at two different ports, the purpose is to perform image mosaicking of these viewpoints videos to obtain a wide visual panoramic video of the operation site.

In traditional image mosaicking, an overlap between images is necessary for generating panoramic image. However, in the case of trocar-retractable cameras, an enough large overlap between cameras is not necessarily preserved during the operation because of trocar movement caused by operation of forceps. Therefore, in this work, feature points tracking in different videos is utilized to increase mosaicking speed and robustness. Moreover, by combining mosaicking and tracking, it is possible to generate panoramic video regardless the overlap between different cameras. The speed and efficiency of the proposed approach is evaluated in this study. From this evaluation, we can deduce that using feature tracking reduces the required number of free view point mosaicking. And then, the computational cost of the whole approach is reduced. Moreover, the mosaicking robustness can be improved.

2 Proposed Method

The general diagram of the proposed mosaicking approach using two cameras is shown in Fig. 2.

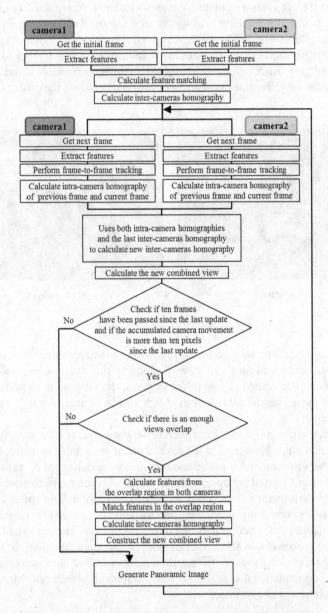

Fig. 2. The general diagram of the proposed mosaicking approach.

At the beginning, an initial panorama image is required. This initial panoramic view is constructed when an enough overlap is found at the exploration time. To construct this view, Speed-Up Robust Feature (SURF) algorithm [9] is utilized to extract feature points from the initial frames acquired from different trocar-retractable cameras. A robust feature matching is then performed by applying a ratio test and double matching from view1 to view2 and vice-verse. Consequently, the inter-cameras homography is calculated from a set of inliers matches found using random sample concise (RANSAC) algorithm [10].

After initialization, continues tracking is performed from frame to frame in each video. In this work, a set of feature points extracted using Good-Feature-to-Track technique [11] are tracked using Pyramidal Lucas-Kanade Optical Flow tracking [12]. These tracked points are utilized to estimate intra-camera homography, which models the relationship of consequent video frames. The current expanded view is then calculated using both intra-camera homographies and the last updated inter-cameras homography. By considering the last updated inter-cameras homography as H_{pano}, the intra-camera homography of the first and second view as H_{view1} and H_{view2}, the current expanded homography view is estimated as in Eq. (1). Figure 3 show an illustration of the estimation process.

$$H_{current} = H_{view1} \times H_{pano} \times H_{view2}^{-1} \tag{1}$$

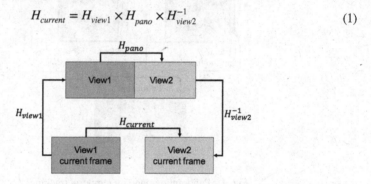

Fig. 3. Estimation of the expanded view.

By using the above mentioned homography estimation methodology, the relationship between different views can be maintained regardless the overlap size. However, the homography error accumulated from frame to frame which cause large estimation error in time. To alleviate this problem and to enhance the overall estimation, an update method is performed if one of the following conditions is satisfied:

(a) The accumulated camera movement is more than 10 pixels since the last update and there is an enough views overlap.
(b) Ten frames have been passed since the last update and there is an enough views overlap.

This update process utilizes the estimated homography to determine the overlap of view1 and view2, and warp the overlap area of view2 to view1 frame. Consequently, the update process is performed using SURF feature points detection and matching.

The matching process is performed locally around the detected points and then the matching time and error are reduced. A correction homography is then calculated from a set of inliers using RANSAC algorithm, and the final corrected homography is calculated as in Eq. (2).

$$H_{final} = H_{correction} * H_{corrent} \tag{2}$$

where, H_{final} is the corrected current expanded view homography, $H_{correction}$ is the correction homography calculated from the overlap area in view1 and view2 and $H_{current}$ is the initial current view estimated homography. The inter-camera homography is now updated using H_{final} and all update conditions are reset.

In the proposed method, it is possible to generate panoramic image using frame-to-frame feature detection and temporal tracking independent of spatial overlap size, as shown in Fig. 4. Also, if there is an enough large overlap between two cameras, we can obtain more accurate panoramic image with direct mosaicking.

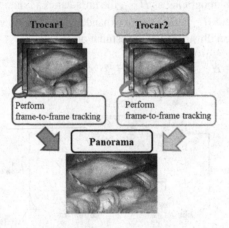

Fig. 4. Panoramic image by temporal tracking.

3   Evaluation Experiments

This section describes the evaluation of the proposed approach. We describe accuracy evaluation of tracking according to camera types and imaging conditions in Sect. 3.1, accuracy evaluation of mosaicking according to overlap size between two cameras in Sect. 3.2. Finally, the comparison of the proposed approach and the conventional mosaicking approach in provided in Sect. 3.3.

All experiments in this study were performed using OpenCV toolkit [13] on a PC with the following specifications; OS is Windows8.1 professional 64 bit, CPU is Intel® Core™ i7-2600 K, RAM is 8 GB, and GPU is NVIDEA GeForce GTX 560 Ti. Moreover, GPU-based features extraction, matching, tracking and image warping were utilized to accelerate the process.

3.1 Tracking Accuracy Evaluation According to Camera Types and Imaging Conditions

In this work, *in vivo* and *in vitro* videos are used to asses feature points tracking accuracy. The trocar-retractable camera is used to capture intra-operational videos of organs which have smooth and specular surfaces. Additionally, a blurring effect may happen during the operation.

3.1.1 Experimental Setup

In this experiment, we use three videos as shown in Fig. 5. These videos are captured at 30 fps for 10 s with a total number of 300 frames. The shelves video shown in Fig. 5(a) is captured by RGB camera (Lumenera Lu170C) which has a resolution of 640 × 480. The intra-operational video of a pig abdomen shown in Fig. 5(b) is captured by trocar camera which has a resolution of 640 × 480, and the intra-operational video shown in Fig. 5(c) is captured with the same trocar camera when blurring and turbulence occurs.

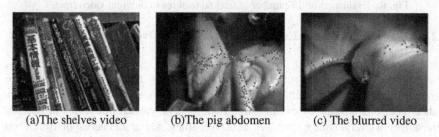

(a)The shelves video   (b)The pig abdomen   (c) The blurred video

Fig. 5. Videos used for tracking accuracy evaluation, blue dots represent the tracked features. (Color figure online)

3.1.2 Results and Discussion

The tracking methodology of the proposed approach is applied to the videos described in the previous section and the results are evaluated. Figure 6 shows the result of feature tracking for all videos. For the video shown in Fig. 5(a), large number of feature points, more than 400, can be always tracked. In comparison with this video, in the intra-operational trocar videos, smaller number of features can be tracked specially in the case of blurred video shown in Fig. 5(c). In this video, the number of tracked features becomes almost 0 when high blurring effect occurs. This fluctuation is caused by noises of video under the influence of using surgical diathermy.

In the proposed approach, intra-camera homography can be calculated if the number of tracked feature points more than seven. Accordingly, we can perform tracking and calculate intra-camera homography in all three videos. However, more accurate intra-camera homography can be calculated when the number of tracked feature points is as large as possible. Therefore, we must examine the feature detection and tracking method for *in vivo* videos in more details.

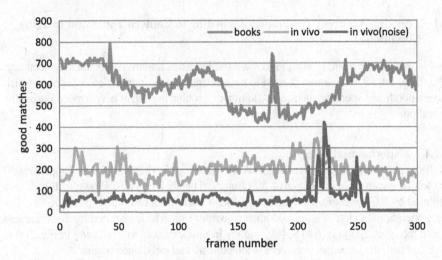

Fig. 6. Evaluation of the number of tracked features in different video frames.

3.2 Mosaicking Accuracy Evaluation According to Overlap Size Between Two Cameras

The proposed approach can maintain the expanded view regardless the overlap size. However, the mosaicking accuracy may be affected by the views overlap size because the update process is affected by overlap size. Therefore, we created test videos of different percentages of overlap range from 20% to 90% of frame size at an interval of 10%. Then, we implement the proposed approach and compare the results using these videos.

3.2.1 Experimental Setup

To create videos for this evaluation, we cut out two 640×480 rectangles from high resolution video captured by the "Stryker 1188 HD" monocular laparoscope, the resolution of which is 1280×720. These rectangles are considered as the viewpoint of camera-1(V_1) and the viewpoint camera-2(V_2), as shown in Fig. 7. The video captured by laparoscope mainly shows serosa of pig stomach. To change the overlap size as a percentage of the whole frame size, we translate V_1 and V_2 in a parallel direction and create eight types of videos, as shown in Table 1.

Table 1. Comparison of mosaicking accuracy for different views overlap size.

Overlap(%)	20	30	40	50	60	70	80	90
Overlap size (# of pixels)	128×480	198×480	256×480	320×480	384×480	448×480	512×480	576×480
Ideal values (X_r, Y_r)	(512, 0)	(448, 0)	(384, 0)	(320, 0)	(256, 0)	(192, 0)	(128, 0)	(64, 0)
Measured values(X_c, Y_c)	(569.9, 16.2)	(483.6, 21.9)	(383.6, −0.4)	(319.6, −0.3)	(255.6, −0.3)	(191.6, −0.4)	(127.6, −0.4)	(63.6, −0.5)
error(pixel)	69.2	49.9	4.5	3.9	3.2	2.5	1.8	1.7

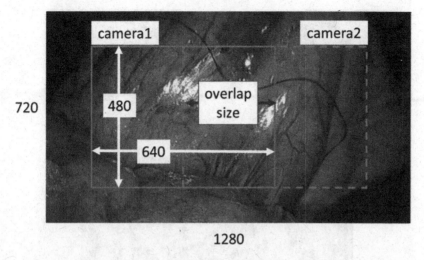

Fig. 7. Evaluation of the number of tracked features in different video frames.

To quantify the accuracy of the estimated panoramic image, we set the central coordinate of V_1 as a relative central position and calculate a relative position of the central coordinate of V_2, regarded as (x, y). We use the error between ideal values (x_r, y_r) and measured values (x_c, y_c) as Euclidean distances for accuracy evaluation as in Eq (3)

$$error = \sqrt{(x_c - x_r)^2 + (y_c - y_r)^2} \qquad (3)$$

3.2.2 Results and Discussion

As noticed from Table 1, the expanded view can be obtained in all cases. However, in the cases of 20% and 30% percentage of overlap, the panoramic image is generated by tracking only and no update is performed. Accordingly, the error is accumulated from frame to frame and the mosaicking accuracy is degraded. In all other cases, when the overlap size is enough for update process, a very good mosaicking accuracy is achieved. Therefore, we deduce that we need to improve the tracking accuracy in order to further improve the mosaicking accuracy specially in the case of small overlap size.

Figure 8(a), (b) shows the viewpoints of camera-1(V_1) and camera-1(V_1) when the overlap size is 40%, and Fig. 8(c) shows the result of mosaicking. We can get very accurate panoramic image. On the other hand, Fig. 8(d) shows a case when errors occur.

Figure 9 shows the error measured for every frame in each video in the interval of 40% to 90% of overlap size. As can be noticed from this figure, the error accumulates between the update process and it is greatly reduced when the update is performed. It is also noticed that, the larger overlap percentages produces higher mosaicking accuracy. The results of this experiment, shows the importance of update process in reducing the accumulated error. However, as the tracking is an important component of the proposed approach, we must analyze of the tracking errors deeply and try other feature detectors in order to improve its accuracy. In this experiment, we only consider the parallel translation. Thus, we have to consider the rotation movement and its accuracy.

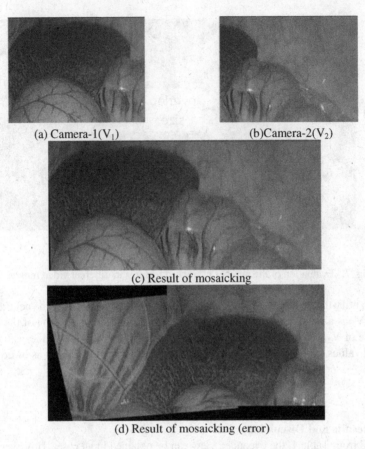

(a) Camera-1(V₁)   (b)Camera-2(V₂)

(c) Result of mosaicking

(d) Result of mosaicking (error)

Fig. 8. Result of mosaicking (overlap size: 40%)

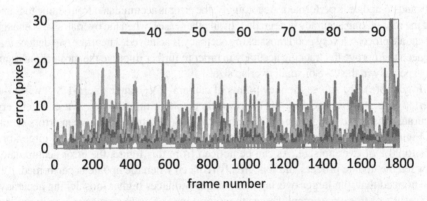

Fig. 9. Comparison of mosaicking accuracy at each video frame.

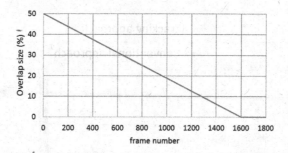

Fig. 10. Changes of the overlap size over video frames.

In addition to the tracking accuracy, physiological motion, forceps motion and tissue deformation would affect the result of mosaicking. We must distinguish these movements from the camera motion in the future.

3.3 Comparison of the Proposed Approach and the Conventional Approach

In conventional image mosaicking approach, an overlap between images is necessary for generating panoramic image. On the other hand, the proposed approach can utilize both tracking and direct mosaicking to generate panoramic image independent of presence of overlap between cameras. To check the efficacy of the proposed approach, we create a video in which the overlap size becomes smaller over time and we perform the comparative evaluation.

3.3.1 Experimental Setup

Similar to 3.3, to create videos for evaluation, we cut out two 640×480 rectangles from a high resolution video captured by the "Stryker 1188 HD" laparoscope. In this experiment, we do not fix the percentages of overlap size; however, we translate V_1 and V_2 while reducing the percentages of overlap, as shown is Fig. 10. The percentages of the overlap size of the first frame is set to 50%, we reduce the percentages at a regular speed until frame number 1600. At the frame number 1600, the percentage of overlap between V_1 and V_2 becomes 0% and we fix V_1 and V_2 until frame number 1800.

We implement the proposed approach and the conventional approach using these videos and the mosaicking accuracy and processing speed are evaluated. We use the error between ideal values (x_r, y_r) and measured values (x_c, y_c) as Euclidean distances for mosaicking accuracy evaluation as in Eq (3).

3.3.2 Results and Discussion

Figure 11 shows the evaluation results of the proposed approach and the conventional approach over time. As can be noticed from this figure, the mosaicking error of the conventional approach is low when an enough overlap is found. However, it becomes unstable from about frame number 1200, and completely stopped at frame number 1400 because of lack of an enough overlap size. On the other hand, the proposed approach can continue the process after frame number 1600 of which percentage of overlap

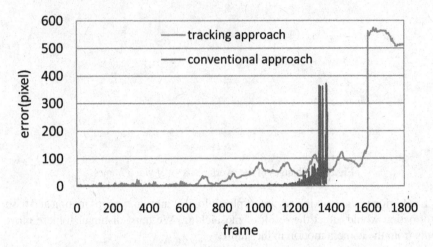

Fig. 11. Comparison proposed approach with conventional approach.

becomes 0%. The error increase from about frame number 800 because of the accumulated error of tracking. Additionally, the proposed approach achieves a frame rate of 18.7 fps while the conventional approach run at 10.1 fps.

From these experiments we deduce that, the proposed approach can provide the expanded view even in the case of 0% overlap, and we can also obtain the advantage in terms of the processing speed.

4   Conclusion

In this work, an approach for abdominal view expansion is proposed. This approach can utilize multiple trocar-retractable camera, image mosaicking and tracking. In contrast to the traditional mosaicking approach, the proposed approach can produce panoramic image even in the case of 0% inter-cameras overlap. Additionally, the proposed approach is about 9 frames per second faster than the conventional approach. The evaluation performed in this work shows that it is difficult to detect the adequate amount of features from trocar camera at the moment; however, the trocar camera is under active development and will be enhanced in the future. Moreover, we found that the overlap size affects the final mosaicking accuracy in the proposed approach. This limitation is mainly caused by the tracking accuracy and we tend to improve the tracking algorithm in the future. In this paper, we used videos created from the laparoscope video; however, we will examine the results using the actual trocar videos in the future.

References

1. Miranda-Luna, R., et al.: Mosaicing of bladder endoscopic image sequences: distortion calibration and registration algorithm. IEEE Trans. Biomed. Eng. **55**(2), 541–553 (2008)
2. Warren, A., et al.: Horizon stabilized—dynamic view expansion for robotic assisted surgery (HS-DVE). Int. J. Comput. Assist. Radiol. and Surg. **7**, 281–288 (2012)

3. Lerotic, M., Chung, A.J., Clark, J., Valibeik, S., Yang, G.-Z.: Dynamic view expansion for enhanced navigation in natural orifice transluminal endoscopic surgery. In: Metaxas, D., Axel, L., Fichtinger, G., Székely, G. (eds.) MICCAI 2008, Part II. LNCS, vol. 5242, pp. 467–475. Springer, Heidelberg (2008)
4. Vemuri, A.S., Liu, K., Ho, Y., Wu, H.: Endoscopic video mosaicing: application to surgery and diagnostics. In: Living Imaging Workshop, 1–2 December, IRCAD, Strasbourg, France (2011)
5. Bergen, T., Ruthotto, S., Munzenmayer, C., Rupp, S., Paulus, D., Winter, C.: Feature-based real-time endoscopic mosaicking. In: Proceeding of 6th International Symposium on Image and Signal Processing and Analysis, pp. 695–700 (2009)
6. Bergen, T., Wittenberg, T.: Stitching and surface reconstruction from endoscopic image sequences: a review of applications and methods. IEEE J. Biomed. Health Inform. 20, 304–321 (2014)
7. Tamadazte, B., Agustinos, A., Cinquin, P., Fiard, G., Voros, S.: Multi-view vision system for laparoscopy surgery. J. Comput. Assist. Radiol. Surg. 10, 195–203 (2015)
8. Okubo, T., Nakaguchi, T., Hayashi, H., Tsumura, T.: Abdominal view expansion by retractable camera. J. Signal Process. 15, 311–314 (2011)
9. Bay, H., Tuytelaars, T., Gool, L.: SURF: speeded up robust features. In: Leonardis, A., Bischof, H., Pinz, A. (eds.) ECCV 2006. LNCS, vol. 3951, pp. 404–417. Springer, Heidelberg (2006). doi:10.1007/11744023_32
10. Fischler, M.A., Bolles, R.C.: Random sample consensus: a paradigm for model fitting with applications to image analysis and automated cartography. Commun. ACM 24, 381–395 (1981)
11. Shi, J., Tomasi, C.: Good features to track. In: 9th IEEE Conference on Computer Vision and Pattern Recognition, pp. 593–600 (1994)
12. Bouguet, J.Y.: Pyramidal implementation of the Lucas Kanade feature tracker: description of the algorithm, Intel Corporation Microprocessor Research Labs (2000)
13. OpenCV 2.4.13.0 documentation (2016). http://docs.opencv.org/2.4/index.html# Accessed 20 June 2016

Assessment of Electromagnetic Tracking Accuracy for Endoscopic Ultrasound

Ester Bonmati[1(✉)], Yipeng Hu[1], Kurinchi Gurusamy[2], Brian Davidson[2],
Stephen P. Pereira[3], Matthew J. Clarkson[1], and Dean C. Barratt[1]

[1] Department of Medical Physics and Biomedical Engineering,
UCL Centre for Medical Image Computing, University College London, London, UK
e.bonmati@ucl.ac.uk
[2] Division of Surgery and Interventional Science, University College London, London, UK
[3] Institute for Liver and Digestive Health, University College London, London, UK

Abstract. Endoscopic ultrasound (EUS) is a minimally-invasive imaging technique that can be technically difficult to perform due to the small field of view and uncertainty in the endoscope position. Electromagnetic (EM) tracking is emerging as an important technology in guiding endoscopic interventions and for training in endotherapy by providing information on endoscope location by fusion with pre-operative images. However, the accuracy of EM tracking could be compromised by the endoscopic ultrasound transducer. In this work, we quantify the precision and accuracy of EM tracking sensors inserted into the working channel of a flexible endoscope, with the ultrasound transducer turned on and off. The EUS device was found to have little (no significant) effect on static tracking accuracy although jitter increased significantly. A significant change in the measured distance between sensors arranged in a fixed geometry was found during a dynamic acquisition. In conclusion, EM tracking accuracy was not found to be significantly affected by the flexible endoscope.

Keywords: Electromagnetic tracking · Endoscopic ultrasound · Image-guided systems · Accuracy · Precision · Validation

1 Introduction

Endoscopic ultrasound (EUS) imaging has become an increasingly important investigative tool in a number of endoscopic procedures, including bronchoscopy, endoscopic procedures involving the gastrointestinal tract, and for localising pancreatic lesions, for example during trans-gastric or trans-duodenal fine needle aspiration (FNA) or during the course of endoscopically guided treatments (endotherapy) [1]. However, many EUS-guided procedures are complex, technically challenging, and require significant experience [2]. The ability to track the 3D position and visualize the endoscope shape, and other surgical instruments inserted through it, in real-time is important for improving

---

M.J. Clarkson and D.C. Barratt—Joint senior author.

© Springer International Publishing AG 2017
T. Peters et al. (Eds.): CARE 2016, LNCS 10170, pp. 36–47, 2017.
DOI: 10.1007/978-3-319-54057-3_4

surgical confidence, reducing the skill required to navigate, and may ultimately allow a less experienced gastroenterologist to perform at an equivalent level as an expert. The additional navigational information becomes especially useful when combined with other diagnostic, planning, and intraoperative imaging modalities, such as pre-operative X-ray computed tomography (CT) or magnetic resonance (MR) images, to provide anatomical context.

Electromagnetic (EM) tracking is arguably the most versatile option for computer-assisted interventions and therapy (CAI) as it allows flexible instruments inside the human body to be tracked in real-time using a very small sensor, and, unlike optical tracking or other image-based tracking methods, it does not require a line-of-sight to be maintained [3]. As a result, EM tracking has rapidly become the tracking method of choice for endoscopic interventions [4], and in turn for EUS-guided procedures [5, 6], and is now incorporated into a number of commercial navigation systems.

Several different protocols have been proposed to evaluate the accuracy of EM tracking systems, mainly to assess static errors [7–11]. The most common approach was proposed by Hummel et al. [8] and has been used to assess new EM systems [12, 13], the accuracy of sensors mounted on US probes [14, 15], and also for optimization [16]. This assessment protocol employs a machined base plate to measure positional and rotational tracking data, offering simplicity, reproducibility, a high precision ground truth and accuracy. This protocol is now widely considered to be the standard method, but there is the limitation that measurement accuracy is a function of translation or rotation [17]. Optical tracking [16] and robots have also been used, however, these solutions are expensive and typically involve complicated calibration procedures [10].

Despite the growing popularity of EM tracking in interventional applications, significant tracking errors due to metallic objects (i.e., steel, aluminium and bronze) placed between the emitter and the sensor, and the use of some electronic devices, such as a C-arm unit, have been reported to cause disturbances to the magnetic field below 4.2 mm [8, 13, 17–20]. Such errors can be particularly prevalent in clinical environments and their sources difficult to control. Therefore, it is challenging to predict the accuracy of an EM tracking system based on measurements from a different environment [21].

The aim of this study was to assess the precision and accuracy of two new EM sensor tools, designed for flexible endoscope tracking, by adapting Hummel et al. standardized protocol specifically for EUS-guided procedures. The main motivation was to determine the accuracy of a widely used EM tracking system when the sensor tools are placed alongside or inside an endoscope working channel, with an EUS probe turned off and on and, to better understand the errors associated with EM instrument tracking in the overall surgical navigation error analysis of EUS-guided procedures.

2 Materials

In this study, we evaluated a NDI Aurora® V3 Tabletop Field Generator (TTFG; Northern Digital, Inc., Waterloo, Ontario, Canada) with a tracking frequency of 40 Hz. This device has shown good performance in terms of accuracy and stability [12], which is required for guiding EUS-related procedures. The TTFG has an ellipsoidal volume of $600 \times 420 \times 600$ mm starting at approximately 120 mm from the physical plane of the board. The manufacturer-reported accuracy of six degrees of freedom (DOFs) sensor tools is 0.80 mm and 0.70° for positional- and rotational data, respectively, in terms of root-mean-square errors (RMSE)[1]. A NDI 6DOF catheter (Type 2) sensor tool, and a NDI 5/6DOF Shape tool (Type 1), were used, both of which are tools designed to be inserted in the working channel of a flexible endoscope. Results reported in this paper are based on tracking data acquired using the NDI Track software included in the NDI ToolBox (version 4.007.007).

To assess the tracking performance of EUS-guided procedures, we used an Aloka ProSound SSD 5000 ultrasound console with an Olympus GF-UCT240 endoscopic ultrasound transducer, operating at a frequency of 11 MHz. The endoscope has a working channel with a diameter of 3.7 mm.

A methacrylate Hummel board [8] with dimensions $550 \times 650 \times 12$ mm was fabricated and used as a ground truth for static measurements. The board contains a grid of 10×12 holes with a precision of 10 μm at a temperature of 20°, spaced 50 mm apart in each direction, and a circle in the centre with 32 holes spaced 11.25° apart, with a radius of 50 mm. To reliably assess the variation along the z-axis of the reference coordinate system, and to enable comparison with older studies, we designed a modular marine plywood platform, which was rigidly secured above the TTFG. This platform allows the board to be easily positioned at three vertical z-levels (120 mm, 220 mm and 320 mm) from the origin of the global coordinate system (see Fig. 1(a)). Two acetal adapters were designed to position tracking tools and endoscopes on the board (see Fig. 1(b–c)). The tracking tool adapters included two pins at a distance of 50 mm that fit into a pair of holes in the board to fix the sensor or endoscope. The endoscope adapter also included four nylon screws to fix the endoscope and avoid undesired rotations or movement. Special attention was paid in using only plastic materials to avoid interference with the field emitted by the TTFG. Based on the tolerances of the fabrication of the phantom, the accuracy of the ground truth setup was estimated to be within 100 μm.

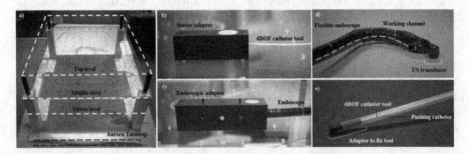

Fig. 1. Experimental setup. (a) The modular platform with 3 positional levels placed above the Aurora Tabletop. (b) Catheter tool sensor attached to the board with the tracking tool adapter. (c) Flexible endoscope attached to the board with the endoscopic adapter. (d) Flexible endoscope with a representation of the working channel. (e) 6DOF catheter tool inserted in the pushing catheter and fixed with the adapter.

---

[1] http://www.ndigital.com/medical/products/aurora/.

3   Methods

3.1   Static Measurements

Using our setup, 72 positions on the grid for each of the three z-levels were available within the ellipsoidal TTFG working volume. For each grid position, 10 s of continuous positional and rotational data were acquired. For the purpose of comparison, measurements were recorded under three different conditions: (a) the sensor in isolation, without the endoscope present (as a reference); (b) the sensor inserted inside the working channel of the endoscope, with the ultrasound console turned off; and (c) the sensor inside the working channel with the ultrasound console and transducer turned on. In order to fix the catheter sensor tool inside the working channel of the flexible endoscope, the tool was first inserted and fixed into a pushing catheter (see Fig. 1(d–e)). Afterwards, the pushing catheter was inserted into the working channel of the endoscope. For the convenience of interpretation of acquired rotational data, the quaternions reported by the tracking system were converted to Euler angles, with rotations about the z-axis being first multiplied when the composite rotation matrices were constructed.

3.2   Precision

Repeated 3D tracking measurements for a static sensor tool contain random errors, commonly referred as *jitter*. For each sample, the Euclidean distance between the measured location and the mean location over all the samples was computed, whilst the rotational distance was calculated as the difference between each measured Euler angle and the mean angle. For each grid position, the precision was quantified by calculating the RMSEs of positional and rotational distances.

3.3   Accuracy

We adapted a distance-based measure to assess the accuracy of tracking based on the TTFG, similar to the one proposed in Hummel protocol [8]. For each grid position, we measured the distance to all of the other ones, which were available, at grid distances of 50 mm, 100 mm and 150 mm as suggested by the protocol (see Fig. 2(a)). The accuracy was calculated as the mean of absolute difference between the ground-truth and the measured distance for each position. This measure provides an indication of how accurate the tracking is when the sensor is moved a certain distance away from a particular reference position. The accuracy along the z-axis, was defined as the mean of the absolute difference in distances between different vertical z-levels (i.e., bottom-middle, middle-top and bottom-top). Estimates of rotational accuracy were obtained by measuring all relative rotations of 11.25°, using the circle included in the board, at the three different levels. In this case, only one rotation was studied due to positioning restrictions of the endoscope adapter.

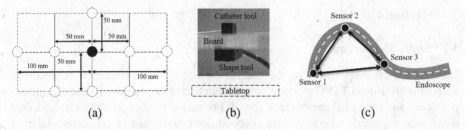

Fig. 2. (a) Illustration of the accuracy measurements in terms of relative distances of 50 mm for rows and columns, and 100 mm for columns. (b) Setup for the EUS-induced distortion error experiment. (c) Position of the sensors inside the working channel to evaluate the dynamic error.

3.4 EUS-Induced Distortion Error

During EUS-guided procedures, the endoscope can be used in conjunction with other sensors to track patient motion and/or other surgical tools. In particular, we were interested in assessing the effect of placing the endoscope between the TTFG and a sensor of interest (in this case, the catheter tool) which may affect the precision and accuracy of the tracking, as both the catheter and endoscope may cause distortion of the magnetic field. In this case, similar to Sects. 3.2 and 3.3 but only for a small grid of 3 × 5 positions in the centre of the board, we first took static measurements without the endoscope (as a reference). We then repeated the experiment having attached the endoscope at the bottom of the board, just at the middle of the 3 × 5 grid positions, using the endoscopic adapter, such that the endoscope remained in a static position between the TTFG and the sensor of interest (see Fig. 2(b)). The grid positions were the closest to the endoscope, thus more likely to affect the tracking accuracy [8, 13, 18–20]. Additionally, the endoscope contained the shape tool in the working channel, and its position was measured as a reference of the distance between the two tracking tools. We then calculated the positional and rotational jitter, and the accuracy as defined in Sects. 3.2 and 3.3.

3.5 Dynamic Errors

To study dynamic error, the 6/5DOF NDI shape tool was inserted into the working channel of the flexible endoscope in a fixed position where the first three sensors (of 7) formed a triangle (see Fig. 2(c)). As a reference, 10 s of data were recorded in a static position and the mean position of each sensor was obtained. The endoscope was manually moved in a random path within the EM working volume while data was acquired continuously for 20 s. For each dynamic measurement, we calculated the distances between each pair of the three sensors which were located in the fixed part of the endoscope. These three distances were then compared with the corresponding mean distances computed from the reference measurements. This measure does not represent the complete "dynamic error" as any errors correlated between sensors, such as those caused by time latency, may cancel out each other. However, this is a simple and useful estimate of the relative dynamic error for applications where relative positions and distances are important, such as the real-time visualisation of the shape of a moving flexible endoscope.

3.6 Statistical Analysis

Paired two-sample Student's t-tests (t-tests), all with standard confidence level $\alpha = 0.05$, were used to compare means of the static precision and accuracy errors between three scenarios (no endoscope, with endoscope and transducer off and with endoscope and transducer on). Additionally, because the errors were based on non-negative distance measures, results from nonparametric Kolmogorov-Smirnov tests (K-S tests) are also reported. In cases where any null hypothesis was rejected, i.e. a statistically significant difference was observed, a one-way analysis of variance (ANOVA) was used to further test if the three population means are likely to be the same. Furthermore, we used a Pearson's linear correlation coefficient (CC) to quantify the linear correlation between errors obtained from these different scenarios, and between the errors and the distance from the sampling location to the reference coordinate origin. Similarly, the t-test, K-S test and CC were used to analyse the EUS-induced distortion errors and the distance errors from dynamic acquisitions, described in Sects. 3.4 and 3.5, respectively, compared to their respective reference measurements.

4 Results

4.1 Precision

Each acquisition of 10 s led to a set of data with more than 400 valid samples. The mean and standard deviation of the positional and rotational jitter, obtained at the three different z-levels, are summarised in Table 1 and Table 2 respectively. Statistically significant difference was found between jitters with no endoscope and when the endoscope's transducer was turned off and on (*p-value* < *0.001* and *p-value* < *0.001*, for t-test and K-S test, respectively). ANOVA also confirmed a statistically significant difference between three errors (*p-value* = *0.025*). Interestingly, positional jitters were correlated with a CC of 0.98 in both cases (both *p-values* < *0.001*). On the other hand, much smaller CCs were observed between rotational jitters (CC = 0.34 and 0.35).

Table 1. Positional jitter averaged for all grid positions, at three different levels, with no endoscope and with the endoscope transducer turned on/off (mean ± STD in mm RMS).

Positional	Lower level	Middle level	Top level
No endoscope	0.01 ± 0.01	0.04 ± 0.01	0.14 ± 0.03
Transducer off	0.01 ± 0.01	0.04 ± 0.01	0.15 ± 0.04
Transducer on	0.02 ± 0.01	0.05 ± 0.01	0.18 ± 0.04

Table 2. Rotational jitter averaged for all grid positions, at three different levels, with no endoscope and with the endoscope transducer turned on/off (mean ± STD in degrees RMS).

Rotational	Lower level	Middle level	Top level
No endoscope	0.02 ± 0.03	0.06 ± 0.03	0.17 ± 0.07
Transducer off	0.12 ± 0.26	0.07 ± 0.03	0.18 ± 0.07
Transducer on	0.33 ± 0.38	0.10 ± 0.05	0.72 ± 0.70

Positional jitters versus Euclidean distance to the origin of the coordinates system is plotted in Fig. 3. A strong correlation was observed between jitters with all CCs greater than 0.89 for measurements from different grid positions and z-levels. Rotational jitters were correlated with the distance to the coordinate's origin with a correlation coefficient of 0.84 when there was no endoscope, a coefficient of 0.30 with the endoscope console turned off and 0.36 with the ultrasound transducer turned on. In this case, the lack of correlation between rotational precision and location was caused by the physical presence of the endoscope

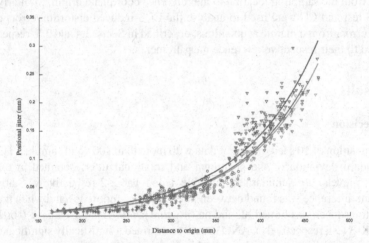

Fig. 3. Positional jitter versus Euclidean distance to origin of the coordinates system (+ = bottom level, o = middle level, ▼ = top level) with the corresponding exponential fitted curves without endoscope (orange), with the ultrasound transducer turned off (green), and with the ultrasound transducer turned on (blue). (Color figure online)

4.2 Accuracy

For each z-level, a total of 52 values in rows and 56 values in columns were available at a distance of 50 mm, 32 values in rows and 40 values in columns were available at a distance of 150 mm, and finally, at a distance of 150 mm, 12 values in rows and 24 values in columns were obtained. Comparisons of the positional mean values are shown in Fig. 4. Overall, no statistically significant difference was found between the positional accuracy without endoscope and with endoscope and the ultrasound transducer on (ANOVA *p-value = 0.496*). Positional accuracies with endoscope and no endoscope were correlated with a Pearson's coefficient higher than 0.81. Additionally, there was no statistically significant difference between the distance from the low level to the top level and the sum of the distances between two adjacent levels ($p\text{-value} = 0.740$, K-S test). Correlation analysis also showed a CC lower than 0.46 between the accuracy of each position and the distance to the origin of the coordinates system in all cases.

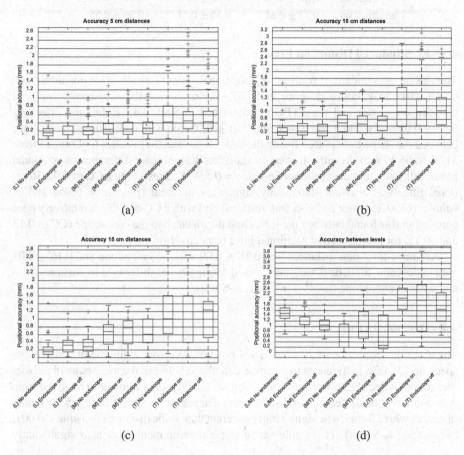

(a)

(b)

(c)

(d)

Fig. 4. Comparison of positional accuracy at a distance of 50 mm (a), 100 mm (b), 150 mm (c), and between levels (d). Boxplots show the absolute difference in distance (median, minimum, maximum, upper and lower quartile) for the bottom (L), middle (M) and top (T) levels.

The rotational accuracy results are summarized in Table 3. Overall, a statistically significant difference was found between the rotational accuracy without endoscope and rotational accuracy with endoscope ($p\text{-value} < 0.001$ and $p\text{-value} < 0.001$, for t-test and K-S test, respectively). However, relatively low CCs were found between the accuracies without endoscope and with endoscope and the transducer on (CCs were 0.49 and 0.46 for the transducer on- and off cases, respectively).

Table 3. Relative rotational error averaged for all 32 positions, at three different levels, with no endoscope and with the endoscope transducer turned on/off (mean ± STD in degrees).

Rotational	Lower level	Middle level	Upper level
No endoscope	0.35 ± 0.48	0.19 ± 0.13	0.21 ± 0.13
Transducer off	0.30 ± 0.36	0.30 ± 0.43	0.47 ± 0.75
Transducer on	0.27 ± 0.31	0.36 ± 0.51	0.39 ± 0.55

4.3 EUS-Induced Distortion Error

The mean ± standard deviation of positional jitter for all grid positions was 0.03 ± 0.01 mm without endoscope, and 0.02 ± 0.00 mm when the endoscope was placed between the sensor and the TTFG (as described in Sect. 3.4). Rotational jitter was 0.05 ± 0.01 mm without endoscope and 0.01 ± 0.00 mm with endoscope. The distance between the shape tool, placed inside the endoscope, and the catheter tool ranged from 31.71 to 65.49 mm. Results showed no statistically significant difference in positional jitters with and without endoscope (*p-value = 0.589*, K-S test) with a CC of 0.92. Rotational jitter was also not statistically significant different (*p-value = 0.962* and *p-value = 0.890*, for t-test and K-S test, respectively) with a CC of 0.76. A relatively poor correlation was found between the jitters and the distance to the endoscope (CC of 0.13 and –0.15, for positional and rotational jitter respectively).

Accuracy for 5 mm distances was 0.18 ± 0.09 with no endoscope and 0.16 ± 0.01 with endoscope. Statistical analysis showed no significant difference in accuracy with and without endoscope (*p-value = 0.862*, K-S test).

4.4 Dynamic Errors

The dynamic acquisition of 20 s led to 894 positional vectors acquired with an average speed of 0.31 m/s. Differences in distance, calculated between the three pairs of sensors (described in Sect. 3.5), were 0.29 ± 0.42 mm, -0.39 ± 0.24 mm and 0.64 ± 0.4 mm. A histogram of the difference in distance between sensors is shown in Fig. 5. Dynamic distances where found to be significantly different than static distances (*p-value < 0.001*, two-sample K-S test). The whole set of static measurements was also significantly

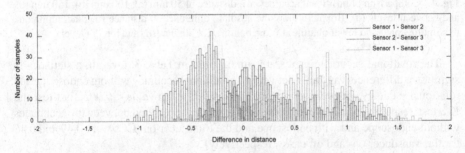

Fig. 5. Histogram of the differences in distance between the three fixed sensors during a dynamic acquisition.

different than the dynamic set of measurements ($p < 0.001$, two-sample t-test). No strong correlation was observed between these three distance errors (CCs were –0.43, –0.18 and 0.09).

5 Discussion

Positional accuracy did not significantly differ using the endoscope and there was no evidence of correlation with the distance to the TTFG. Our analysis shows clear evidence that the error obtained, when moving along the z-axis (away from the emitter), is cumulative. This effect was also observed with no endoscope. This error appears to be systematic, thus, should be taken into account and corrected if possible. Rotational accuracy was also not strongly correlated with the distance to origin. Due to the limitation of the endoscopic adapter, only rotation about the Z axis was evaluated. This limitation may be overcome by creating two more adapters that allow rotation of the endoscope on the other two axes. On the other hand, positional jitter was found to significantly increase when the sensor was inserted in the working channel of the endoscope and was positively correlated with the distance to the origin of the coordinates system, remaining below 0.2 mm for all cases. Rotational jitter also increased, with a precision error of 0.7° in the worst case. In this case, no evidence was found regarding the correlation with the distance to the origin of the coordinates system.

EUS-induced distortion error was measured with the endoscope between the sensor and the TTFG. Our results showed no evidence of significant distortion when the endoscope was placed between 32 and 65 mm to the sensor. These positions were the closest on the grid to the endoscope during the experiments and therefore more likely to affect the accuracy. Thus, tracking other objects, such as clinical instruments, in combination with EUS seems feasible, although the accuracy of electromagnetic tracking should be quantified with the instrument of interest.

Errors introduced when the sensor is moving are of interest, although these have not been included in most assessment protocols reported in the literature [11]. In this work, we assessed a simple distance-based relative error between sensors during a dynamic acquisition, which was found to change significantly, with all mean errors below 0.7 mm. The dynamic error may affect the position and shape displayed of the flexible endoscopes during guidance, and its clinical impact will be dependent on the application.

The robustness of tracking accuracy with respect to the use of an endoscope was assessed by repeating the measurements with the EUS probe turned off and on, and without the endoscope being present. It is worth mentioning that the experiments were performed in a laboratory where conditions may differ from a clinical interventional suite, as the presence of other devices, such as a C-arm, may interfere in the measurements. To the best of our knowledge, no endoscope for EUS-guided procedures with an integrated EM sensor currently exists, although similar devices are available for bronchoscopy [22] and colonoscopy [23]. In addition, having the sensor tool inserted in the working channel has the advantages of portability and compatibility across different endoscope models and manufacturers compared with permanently embedding sensors within the wall of the flexible and/or bending sections. Our results suggest that it is possible to combine EUS and EM tracking without compromising the tracking accuracy significantly, although further research is required to estimate localisation errors for instruments, such as needle-tips, for specific clinical applications, which are likely to have different accuracy requirements.

This work focused on the study of static errors (jitter and relative accuracy), and partial distance-based dynamic errors, as we believe they are the main errors affecting the application of interest in EUS-guided procedures.

6 Conclusions

In this paper, we present the first accuracy study of 6DOF EM tracking tools inserted into the working channel of an endoscopic ultrasound probe, by using and extending a standardized protocol. Accuracy was not found to be highly affected by the endoscope for EUS-guided procedures, although the jitter increased. Future work includes evaluation of the tools in an interventional suite using different endoscopes as well as an assessment of the shape provided by the shape tool inserted in an endoscope.

Acknowledgment. This publication presents independent research supported by Cancer Research UK (CRUK) (Multidisciplinary Award C28070/A19985).

The authors would like to thank Joe Evans from the UCL department of Medical Physics and Biomedical Engineering for making and helping to design the accuracy assessment board, the supporting structures, and adapters.

References

1. Williams, D.B., Sahai, A.V., Aabakken, L., Penman, I.D., van Velse, A., Webb, J., Wilson, M., Hoffman, B.J., Hawes, R.H.: Endoscopic ultrasound guided fine needle aspiration biopsy: a large single centre experience. Gut **44**, 720–726 (1999)
2. Mertz, H., Gautam, S.: The learning curve for EUS-guided FNA of pancreatic cancer. Gastrointest. Endosc. **59**, 33–37 (2004)
3. Mori, K., Deguchi, D., Sugiyama, J., Suenaga, Y., Toriwaki, J., Maurer, C.R., Takabatake, H., Natori, H.: Tracking of a bronchoscope using epipolar geometry analysis and intensity-based image registration of real and virtual endoscopic images. Med. Image Anal. **6**, 321–336 (2002)
4. Fried, M.P., Kleefield, J., Gopal, H., Reardon, E., Ho, B.T., Kuhn, F.A.: Image-guided endoscopic surgery: results of accuracy and performance in a multicenter clinical study using an electromagnetic tracking system. Laryngoscope **107**, 594–601 (1997)
5. Sumiyama, K., Suzuki, N., Kakutani, H., Hino, S., Tajiri, H., Suzuki, H., Aoki, T.: A novel 3-dimensional EUS technique for real-time visualization of the volume data reconstruction process. Gastrointest. Endosc. **55**, 723–728 (2002)
6. Fritscher-Ravens, A., Knoefel, W.T., Krause, C., Swain, C.P., Brandt, L., Patel, K.: Three-dimensional linear endoscopic ultrasound—feasibility of a novel technique applied for the detection of vessel involvement of pancreatic masses. Am. J. Gastroenterol. **100**, 1296–1302 (2005)
7. Frantz, D.D., Wiles, A.D., Leis, S.E., Kirsch, S.R.: Accuracy assessment protocols for electromagnetic tracking systems. Phys. Med. Biol. **48**, 2241–2251 (2003)

8. Hummel, J.B., Bax, M.R., Figl, M.L., Kang, Y., Maurer, C., Birkfellner, W.W., Bergmann, H., Shahidi, R.: Design and application of an assessment protocol for electromagnetic tracking systems. Med. Phys. **32**, 2371–2379 (2005)

9. Wilson, E., Yaniv, Z., Zhang, H., Nafis, C., Shen, E., Shechter, G., Wiles, A.D., Peters, T., Lindisch, D., Cleary, K.: A hardware and software protocol for the evaluation of electromagnetic tracker accuracy in the clinical environment: a multi-center study. In: Proceedings of SPIE, vol. 6509, pp. 65092T–65092T–11 (2007)

10. Nagy, M.: Towards unified electromagnetic tracking system assessment — static errors. IEEE Eng. Med. Biol. Mag. **236**, 1905–1908 (2011)

11. Franz, A.M., Haidegger, T., Birkfellner, W., Cleary, K., Peters, T.M., Maier-Hein, L.: Electromagnetic tracking in medicine - A review of technology, validation, and applications. IEEE Trans. Med. Imaging **33**, 1702–1725 (2014)

12. Maier-Hein, L., Franz, A.M., Birkfellner, W., Hummel, J., Gergel, I., Wegner, I., Meinzer, H.P.: Standardized assessment of new electromagnetic field generators in an interventional radiology setting. Med. Phys. **39**, 3424–3434 (2012)

13. Franz, A.M., Schmitt, D., Seitel, A., Chatrasingh, M., Echner, G., Oelfke, U., Nill, S., Birkfellner, W., Maier-Hein, L.: Standardized accuracy assessment of the calypso wireless transponder tracking system. Phys. Med. Biol. **59**, 6797–6810 (2014)

14. Franz, A.M., März, K., Hummel, J., Birkfellner, W., Bendl, R., Delorme, S., Schlemmer, H.P., Meinzer, H.P., Maier-Hein, L.: Electromagnetic tracking for US-guided interventions: standardized assessment of a new compact field generator. Int. J. Comput. Assist. Radiol. Surg. **7**, 813–818 (2012)

15. Hastenteufel, M., Vetter, M., Meinzer, H.P., Wolf, I.: Effect of 3D ultrasound probes on the accuracy of electromagnetic tracking systems. Ultrasound Med. Biol. **32**, 1359–1368 (2006)

16. Qi, Y., Sadjadi, H., Yeo, C.T., Hashtrudi-zaad, K., Member, S., Fichtinger, G.: Electromagnetic tracking performance analysis and optimization, pp. 6534–6538 (2014)

17. Lugez, E., Sadjadi, H., Pichora, D.R., Ellis, R.E., Akl, S.G., Fichtinger, G.: Electromagnetic tracking in surgical and interventional environments: usability study. Int. J. Comput. Assist. Radiol. Surg. **10**, 253–262 (2015)

18. Hummel, J., Figl, M., Kollmann, C., Bergmann, H., Birkfellner, W.: Evaluation of a miniature electromagnetic position tracker. Med. Phys. **29**, 2205–2212 (2002)

19. Nixon, M.A., McCallum, B.C., Fright, W.R., Price, N.B.: The effects of metals and interfering fields on electromagnetic trackers. Presence Teleoperators Virtual Environ. **7**, 204–218 (1998)

20. Kirsch, S.R., Schilling, C., Brunner, G.: Assesment of metallic distortions of an electromagnetic tracking system. In: SPIE Medical Imaging. International Society for Optics and Photonics (2006)

21. Yaniv, Z., Wilson, E., Lindisch, D., Cleary, K.: Electromagnetic tracking in the clinical environment. Med. Phys. **36**, 876–892 (2009)

22. Leong, S., Ju, H., Marshall, H., Bowman, R., Yang, I., Ree, A.-M., Saxon, C., Fong, K.M.: Electromagnetic navigation bronchoscopy: a descriptive analysis. J. Thorac. Dis. **4**, 173–185 (2012)

23. Szura, M., Bucki, K., Matyja, A., Kulig, J.: Evaluation of magnetic scope navigation in screening endoscopic examination of colorectal cancer. Surg. Endosc. **26**, 632–638 (2012)

Extended Multi-resolution Local Patterns - A Discriminative Feature Learning Approach for Colonoscopy Image Classification

Siyamalan Manivannan[✉] and Emanuele Trucco

CVIP, School of Science and Engineering (Computing),
University of Dundee, Dundee, UK
smanivannan@dundee.ac.uk

Abstract. We propose a novel local image descriptor called the *Extended Multi-resolution Local Patterns*, and a discriminative probabilistic framework for learning its parameters together with a multi-class image classifier. Our approach uses training data with image-level labels to learn the features which are discriminative for multi-class colonoscopy image classification. Experiments on a three class (abnormal, normal, uninformative) white-light colonoscopy image dataset with 2800 images show that the proposed feature perform better than popular hand-designed features used in the medical as well as in the computer vision literature for image classification.

1 Introduction

More than one million new Colorectal cancer (CRC) cases are diagnosed yearly worldwide, and CRC remains the third leading cause of cancer death in the world [1]. There is compelling evidence that removing adenomas from the colon substantially reduces the risk of a patient developing CRC [1]. If CRC is diagnosed in its earliest stages, the chance of survival is 90% [1]. Clearly, early identification of colonic abnormalities is crucially important.

Adenoma detection rate (ADR) is a commonly used predictor of the risk of developing CRC after undergoing a colonoscopy screening [2]. Although colonoscopy remains the gold standard for CRC screening, CRC miss rate has been reported as high as 6% [3], posing risk of developing colon cancer due to a failure to detect treatable lesions in time. It is therefore arguable that a reliable computer-aided detection system specialised for identifying suspicious colonic abnormalities in colonoscopy videos could contribute to improve ADR, e.g. by presenting clinicians with a second opinion obtained by objective and repeatable methods.

In this paper we propose an automated system to classify colonoscopy images into three classes: abnormal, normal and uninformative. The abnormal images contain various abnormalities such as polyps, cancers, ulcers and bleeding, appearing in a variety of sizes, positions and orientations in the image. The normal images contain none and show a clear healthy colon wall. The uninformative images contain images which are blurred due to out of focus (e.g., camera

© Springer International Publishing AG 2017
T. Peters et al. (Eds.): CARE 2016, LNCS 10170, pp. 48–58, 2017.
DOI: 10.1007/978-3-319-54057-3_5

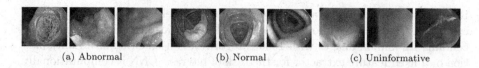

(a) Abnormal   (b) Normal   (c) Uninformative

Fig. 1. Example images from our dataset.

pushed against the colon wall) or sharp camera movements. Note that we are not specifically interested in detecting uninformative frames as done in the existing approaches (e.g. [4]), but our target is a multi-class colonoscopy image classification (Fig. 1).

Various hand-designed features (e.g. SIFT) have been explored for colonoscopy image classification (discussed in Sect. 2). However, these features may not be optimally discriminative for classifying images from particular domains (e.g. colonoscopy), as not necessarily tuned to the domain's characteristics. We instead propose a learning approach, which jointly learns discriminative local features together with a multi-class image classifier using training data with image-level labels. Since our features are learned from the data we expect them to be more discriminative than hand-designed ones. Comparative experiments with our colonoscopy dataset show that the learned features perform better than popular features used in the medical as well in the computer vision literature for image classification.

2   Related Work

The approaches proposed for colonoscopy image analysis are mainly focussed on identifying appropriate features; various hand-crafted features such as color wavelet co-variance (CWC) [5], color histograms (CH) [6], gray-level co-occurrence matrices (GLCM) [7], Root-SIFT (rSIFT) [8], Local Binary Patterns (LBP) [8], Local Ternary Patterns (LTP) [8] have been explored. For example, LBP and GLCM for normal/abnormal classification [7,8], CWC for polyp detection [5], and for classification [7].

Feature learning approaches, e.g. [9–11], on the other hand, learn domain-specific discriminative local features and report improved performance compared to hand-crafted features in various applications, e.g. medical image segmentation [9], and natural image retrieval [11,12]. However, these approaches require a labelled dataset for learning; e.g., Becker et al. [9] uses manual region-level segmentations to learn filters for curvilinear structure segmentation in retinal and microscopy images.

Convolutional neural nets (CNN) have been widely used to jointly learn features and a classifier. Usually CNN requires a large amount of training data [13]; when this is not available, CNN may give worse performance than traditional, hand-crafted features with feature encoding methods such as *sparse coding* [13].

Recently, transfer learning approaches have been widely used (e.g. [14]) to overcome this, where a CNN model trained on a large dataset (e.g. ImageNet, which contains 1.2 million images with 1000 categories), is used either as an initialization or a fixed feature extractor for the task of interest. CNN is computationally expensive to train, even on the GPU [15].

Since obtaining region-level annotations (to learn features as in [9–11]) is a difficult, time-consuming task, we propose a feature learning approach which uses only the image-level labels. Requiring image-labels instead of region-level labels makes annotations less expensive, hence more feasible in practice. Compared to CNN, our approach does not require pre-training on large dataset, or specialized hardware such as GPU for training.

3   Method

First we introduce our notation, and then we define the structure of our feature in Sect. 3.1. Section 3.2 proposes the learning algorithm to learn the parameters of the feature together with a multi-class image classifier. We call the learned feature *Extended Multi-Resolution Local Patterns* (xMRLP).

We characterize an image I_i by a set of local features $\{\mathbf{x}_{ij}\}_{j=1}^{N_i}$, where N_i is the number of local features in I_i. Let's consider the general case of labels, whereby an image is associated with an image-level soft label indicating, for e.g., class probabilities. Our goal is to learn the parameters of the xMRLP features as well as a multi-class classifier based on the given training data, which is formed by the set of tuples $\mathcal{D} = \{(I_i, \tilde{P}_i)\}_{i=1}^{M}$, where M is the number of images in $\mathcal{D}$, and $\tilde{P}_i \in [0,1]^C$ corresponds to a C-dimensional vector of soft labels of the ith training image associated with the C classes. We assume that $\sum_{c=1}^{C} \tilde{P}(y_i = c) = 1$, where $\tilde{P}(y_i = c)$ is the latent class assignment of the image I_i to class c.

3.1   Extended Multi-resolution Local Patterns

Let I_{ij} be the intensity of the jth pixel in the ith image. To capture local context and to make the descriptor less sensitive to noise, we use the sampling pattern widely adopted in feature descriptors e.g. [16]. Figure 2 shows a 3-resolution version of the sampling pattern, where the local neighbourhood around the jth pixel of image I_i is quantized at three resolution levels. Eight sampling points are considered at each resolution. At each sampling point, a Gaussian filter with standard deviation proportional to the size of the support region (circle around each sampling point in Fig. 2) is applied to collect information from that region.

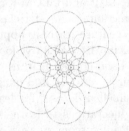

Fig. 2. An example sampling pattern.

Let I_{ij}^s, $s = 1, \ldots, d$, represents the intensity value at the s-th sampling point in the pattern around the jth pixel of image I_i (e.g. $d = 24$ in Fig. 2). We define

$\mathbf{x}_{ij} \in \mathbb{R}^d$ as the xMRLP descriptor vector at pixel j in image I_i using the multi-resolution sampling pattern with d sampling points:

$$\mathbf{x}_{ij}(\boldsymbol{a}) = \left[I_{ij} - a_1 I_{ij}^1, \ldots, I_{ij} - a_d I_{ij}^d \right] \tag{1}$$

where $\boldsymbol{a} = [a_1, \ldots, a_d]$ defines the weights for different neighbourhood regions.

Note that, xMRLP is an improved version of the *Multi-resolution Local Patterns* (MRLP) descriptor proposed in [17,18] for cell image classification. In MRLP the weights for the local neighborhoods were fixed to 1, i.e. $a_i = 1, \forall i$ (Eq. 1).

3.2 A Discriminative Multi-class Framework for Learning

In this section we propose a discriminative framework based on *image-to-class distances* (I2CD) [19] to jointly learn the feature parameter ($\boldsymbol{a}$ in Eq. 1) and an image-level multi-class probabilistic classifier for colonoscopy image classification.

Image to Class Distances. The I2CD was first introduced by Boiman et al. [19] in the NBNN classifier. It requires no training phase, and classifies an image by comparing its distance to different classes. A relaxed version of I2CD was proposed in [20], showing improved performance over the original version for complex datasets. The relaxed version of I2CD is given as:

$$D_{ic}(\boldsymbol{a}) = \frac{1}{N_i P} \sum_{j=1}^{N_i} \sum_{p=1}^{P} \| \mathbf{x}_{ij} - \mathbf{x}_{ij}^{cp} \|_2^2 \tag{2}$$

where $\mathbf{x}_{ij}^{cp}$ is the pth nearest neighbour of $\mathbf{x}_{ij}$ in the cth class, P is the number of considered neighbours. In all the reported experiments we set $P = 3$.

Discriminative Probabilistic Softmax Classifier. Equation (3) below defines a discriminative probabilistic classifier. This classifier outputs the posterior probability of an image I_i belonging to a class c based on the I2CD.

$$P(y_i = c | \{\mathbf{x}_{ij}\}) = \frac{\exp^{-\gamma_c D_{ic}}}{\sum_{l=1}^{C} \exp^{-\gamma_l D_{il}}} \tag{3}$$

The class c maximising the probability above is the one associated with the smallest I2CD over all classes. In Eq. (3) $\{\gamma_l\}_{l=1}^C$ are the classifier parameters.

The Objective Function. Equation (4) defines the objective function to learn the feature parameter $\boldsymbol{a}$ and the classifier parameters $\{\gamma_l\}_{l=1}^C$.

$$\mathcal{L}(\boldsymbol{a}, \{\gamma_l\}_{l=1}^C) = -\frac{1}{M} \sum_{i=1}^{M} \sum_{l=1}^{C} \tilde{P}(y_i = l) \log \left(P(y_i = l | \{\mathbf{x}_{ij}\}) \right) + \beta \| \boldsymbol{a} + \mathbf{1} \|_2^2 \tag{4}$$

where, the first term maximizes the target posterior probabilities of the images in the training set and second term is a regularisation term, prevents the parameters a from becoming arbitrary high and makes their values close to -1 (as in MRLP). We set $\beta = 1$ for all the reported experiments.

We use a coordinate descent method to optimize Eq. (4), where we learn one parameter at a time while keeping the others constant.

Note that, learning the feature parameters is similar to *metric learning* approaches. For example in [21], class-specific distance metrices were learned to compare images with different classes, and the class which gives the smallest I2CD was considered as the target class for that image. However, in Sect. 4.2 we show that the learned features when they are combined with the traditional feature encoding methods such as sparse coding and a SVM classifier performs better than directly using them (as in [21]).

4   Experiments

This section reports our comparative experiments and the results based on the xMRLP descriptor and other features such as LBP, LTP, rSIFT, RP.

Materials: We collected 82 white-light colonoscopy video segments from the Internet. K-means clustering was applied to select a representative subset of images from each video segment based on color statistics (mean, std, skewness and entropy in RGB color chennels) and texture features (LBP histograms). From each video one frame per cluster was randomly selected and annotated by a clinical expert who provided image-level annotations. It is observed that the movement of the colonoscope is fast in normal videos compared to the abnormal ones as the corresponding colon segments do not need a careful inspection of the colonic walls. Therefore the number of clusters for a video v_i was experimentally set to $\frac{V}{7}$ for normal and $\frac{V}{10}$ for abnormal videos, where V is the total number of images in v_i. The final dataset contains 1000 abnormal, 900 normal and 900 uninformative images. All images in the final dataset are rescaled preserving the aspect ratio so that the maximum dimension (row or column) of each image is 300 pixels.

Experimental setup and evaluation criteria: All the local features are extracted from RGB color patches of size $3 \times 16 \times 16$ with an overlap of Q pixels in vertical and horizontal directions. The sampling pattern shown in Fig. 2 (3 resolution, 8 sampling points in each resolution) is used for xMRLP, LBP and LTP features. We rescale the sampling pattern such that all the sampling points lie inside the 16×16 image patches.

The classification performance is measured as the average of the per-class accuracies (mean-class accuracies, MCA) measured on the test test. All the experiments were repeated 10 times and the MCA averaged over these iterations are reported. In each run we randomly selected 300 images from each class for training and use the rest for testing.

Table 1. Performance of various features using the softmax classifier (Eq. 3).

Feature	rSIFT	RP	MRLP	xMRLP (proposed)
Feature dimensionality	384	200	72	**72**
MCA	82.83 ± 1.20	84.37 ± 0.48	80.97 ± 0.92	**87.07 ± 0.40**

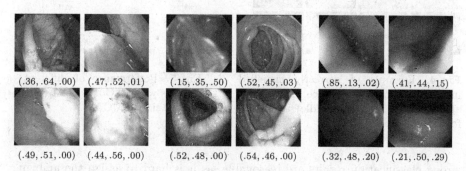

| (.36, .64, .00) | (.47, .52, .01) | (.15, .35, .50) | (.52, .45, .03) | (.85, .13, .02) | (.41, .44, .15) |
| (.49, .51, .00) | (.44, .56, .00) | (.52, .48, .00) | (.54, .46, .00) | (.32, .48, .20) | (.21, .50, .29) |

Fig. 3. Example of wrongly classified images (abnormal - first two columns, normal - next two columns, uninformative - last two columns) and their confidence values using the xMRLP features. The values in the brackets are correspond to $P(y = \text{abnormal})$, $P(y = \text{normal})$ and $P(y = \text{uninfomative})$ respectively.

4.1 Effect of Feature Learning

This section compares the xMRLP feature with baseline features rSIFT, RP and MRLP.

For each feature the representation of a patch was obtained by concatenating the features extracted from each of the color channels of the RGB color space. This led to a dimensionality of 72 (3 colors $\times$ 3 resolutions $\times$ 8 sampling points) for MRLP and xMRLP, and 3×128 for rSIFT. Each of the vectorized color patch of dimension $3 \times 16 \times 16$ is projected to a compressed space of dimension 200 using a random projection matrix [22] to get a RP feature.

In the feature learning stage of xMRLP we use only 50 images from each of the 3 classes, since the I2CD calculations are computationally expensive due to nearest neighbour search. In the classification stage we randomly sample 50,000 local features from each class of the training images and calculate the I2CD between a test image and the training set to do the classification. In both cases features are extracted densely without overlap ($Q = 0$).

Table 1 compares the performance of different features; xMRLP improves the performance of MRLP by about 7%, suggesting that learning can capture discriminative information. xMRLP also outperforms rSIFT and RP with low dimensional representation, makes the I2CD classifier computationally efficient.

Since the proposed framework can also provide probabilistic outputs for the test images, Figs. 3 and 4 show example of the wrongly and correctly classified test images and their confidence values based on the probabilistic soft-max classifier given in Eq. (3). As can be seen from Fig. 3 the probability outputs and the

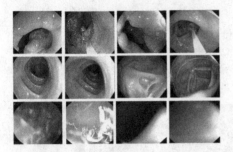

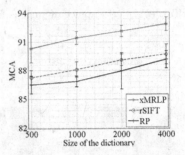

Fig. 4. Example of correctly classified images with high confidence ($P > 0.9$). abnormal(top), normal(middle) and uninformative(bottom).

Fig. 5. Performance of different features with LLC and SVM (dictionary size vs MCA).

wrong classification results are reasonable, as it is hard to assign the ambiguous images (i.e. images with ambiguous appearance) to a single class with high confidence.

4.2   XMRLP with Feature Encoding and SVM Classifier

The softmax classifier used in Sect. 4.1 is computationally expensive due to the nearest neighbour search involved in the I2CD calculations. Feature encoding methods (e.g. [23]) with SVM classifier, on the other hand, are widely used in medical image analysis [8] and are computationally efficient compared to I2CD calculations. Therefore, in this section we evaluate the performance of the learned xMRLP features (after learning them as explained in Sect. 4.1) using a feature encoding method called *Locality Constraint Linear Coding* (LLC) [23] and a SVM classifier. We show that xMRLP features with LCC+SVM perform better than other features as well as xMRLP features with the soft-max classifier (Sect. 4.1).

Since feature encoding is computationally efficient, we extracted features more densely, with an overlap of $Q = 12$ pixels. For each feature type we randomly sampled 100,000 local features to learn the dictionary using k-means. We used SVM classifier (LIBSVM [24]) with an exponential χ^2 kernel and report the performance in Fig. 5. xMRLP feature outperforms other features even with a smaller dictionary size (500) suggesting that learned features are better than other features considered. When the dictionary size is 4000, xMRLP gives a MCA of 92.8% which is better than the MCA obtained by rSIFT (89.7%) and RP (89.1%).

4.3   Comparison with the Features Proposed for Colonoscopy

This section compares the performance of various features proposed for colonoscopy image classification literature such as LBP [8], LTP [8], color his-

Table 2. Performance of different features (S -size of the image representation).

Feat	CH	CWC	CWC2	GLCM	WGLCM	LBP	LTP	rSIFT	RP	MRLP	xMRLP
S	225	216	240	144	144	531	1062	4000	4000	4000	4000
MCA	85.0	79.3	79.7	80.1	83.0	87.4	89.6	89.7	89.1	91.3	**92.8**
std($\pm$)	1.17	0.8	0.8	0.87	0.5	0.52	0.72	1.05	0.90	0.8	**0.70**

tograms (CH) [6], GLCM [25], GLCM on wavelet images (WGLCM) [26], CWC [5] and CWC with higher-order statistics (CWC2) [7].

For LBP and LTP features we use a three resolution version of the sampling patterns as explained in Sect. 4. These features are extracted with an overlap of $Q = 12$ pixels. The LTP parameters were learned from a 5-fold cross validation on the training set. To make a fair comparison we used the same SVM classifier with an exponential χ^2 kernel for this experiment.

The results are reported in Table 2. The proposed xMRLP feature outperforms others by a large margin. xMRLP feature takes about 0.3 s to classify an image compared to 1.1 s and 1.3 s by RP and rSIFT features respectively on an Intel Core-i7 machine with 8 GB RAM. These times include the time for feature extraction and encoding with a dictionary of size 1000.

4.4 Comparison with Deep Convolutional Neural Nets

Since CNN was widely applied for bio-medical [27] as well in non-medical [13] applications, the following experiments were done with CNN to evaluate its performance on our colonoscopy dataset.

Training using colon dataset: A shallow network (Fig. 6) was trained (from scratch) using only the images from the colon dataset with data augmentation (mirrored images). This network gives an MCA of 76.1±0.7%, which is ~15% less compared to our approach (92.8%). This is mainly due to the lack of data used for training. Similar findings were reported in [13] on the Caltech101 dataset[1]; CNN trained on this dataset gives an accuracy of 46%, compared to the accuracy of 84% obtained by the hand-designed features with feature encoding.

Transfer learning: In this experiment we fine-tuned the ImageNet (1.2 Million images) trained model "AlexNet" [15] using the colon dataset with data augmentation (mirrored images, and randomly cropped image regions of size 227×227 from images of size 256×256). This fine-tuned net gives a MCA of 92.9 ± 0.6%, which is similar to the MCA obtained by our approach (92.8%).

Unlike our approach, CNN is designed to capture features at multiple scales. Therefore, the classification performance of CNN can be expected to be high compared to our approach. However this ImageNet pretrained CNN shows similar performance compared to our approach, as the results on this dataset are saturated at ~93%. Although results are similar, our approach does not require

---

[1] http://www.vision.caltech.edu/Image_Datasets/Caltech101/.

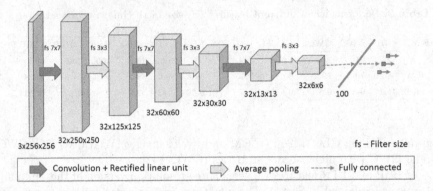

Fig. 6. The shallow CNN architecture used for the colonoscopy image classification.

a larger dataset for pre-training or higher computational power such as GPU. Our approach takes ∼1.5 h to train on a CPU with our unoptimized Matlab code on an Intel Core-i7 machine with 8 GB RAM compared to ∼20 min fine-tuning time required by CNN on NVidia Tesla K40 GPU[2] with 12 GB RAM.

For the above two experiments we use the following parameters to train the network: learning rate 10^{-4}, momentum 0.9, weight decay 5×10^{-4}. The maximum number of iterations were set to 10000 and 7000 for the first and second experiments respectively. The library Caffe [28] was used in all the CNN-related experiments.

5   Conclusions

We presented a novel discriminative feature learning approach for multi-class colonoscopy image classification, which jointly learns the parameters of the proposed xMRLP features together with an image-level classifier using training data with image-level labels. Various comparative experiments on a colonoscopy dataset with the features proposed in the literature of colonoscopy as well as computer vision show that our learned features outperform others. The proposed approach is not restricted to colonoscopy images, hence our future work will explore applications to other medical image domains.

References

1. Atkin, W., Cook, C., Cuzick, J., Edwards, R., Northover, J., Wardle, J.: Once-only flexible sigmoidoscopy screening in prevention of colorectal cancer: a multicentre randomised controlled trial. Lancet **132**, 1624–1633 (2010)
2. Wallace, M.: Improving colorectal adenoma detection: technology or technique? Gastroenterology **132**, 1221–1223 (2007)

---

[2] Tesla K40 GPU used for this research was donated by the NVIDIA Corporation.

3. Bressler, B., Paszat, L.F., Chen, Z., Rothwell, D.M., Vinden, C., Rabeneck, L.: Rates of new or missed colorectal cancers after colonoscopy and their risk factors: a population-based analysis. Gastroenterology **132**(1), 96–102 (2007)

4. Arnold, M., Ghosh, A., Lacey, G., Patchett, S., Mulcahy, H.: Indistinct frame detection in colonoscopy videos. In: Machine Vision and Image Processing Conference, pp. 47–52(2009)

5. Karkanis, S.A., Iakovvidis, D.K., Maroulis, D.E., Karras, D.A., Tzivras, M.: Computer aided tumor detection in endoscopic video using color wavelet features. IEEE Trans. IT Biomed. **7**, 141–152 (2003)

6. Khun, P.C., Zhuo, Z., Yang, L.Z., Liyuan, L., Jiang, L.: Feature selection and classification for wireless capsule endoscopic frames. In: Biomedical and Pharmaceutical Engineering, pp. 1–6 (2009)

7. Lima, C., Barbosa, D., Ramos, A., Tavares, A., Montero, L., Carvalho, L.: Classification of endoscopic capsule images by using color wavelet features, higher order statistics and radial basis functions. In: IEEE Engineering in Medicine and Biology Society, pp. 1242–1245 (2008)

8. Manivannan, S., Wang, R., Trucco, E., Hood, A.: Automatic normal-abnormal video frame classification for colonoscopy. In: IEEE International Symposium on Biomedical Imaging, pp. 644–647 (2013)

9. Becker, C.J., Rigamonti, R., Lepetit, V., Fua, P.: Supervised feature learning for curvilinear structure segmentation. In: Medical Image Computing and Computer-Assisted Intervention, pp. 526–533 (2013)

10. Brown, M., Hua, G., Winder, S.: Discriminative learning of local image descriptors. IEEE Pattern Anal. Mach. Intell. **33**, 43–57 (2011)

11. Simonyan, K., Vedaldi, A., Zisserman, A.: Learning local feature descriptors using convex optimisation. IEEE Pattern Anal. Mach. Intell. **36**, 1573–1585 (2014)

12. Philbin, J., Isard, M., Sivic, J., Zisserman, A.: Descriptor learning for efficient retrieval. In: European Conference on Computer Vision, pp. 677–691 (2010)

13. Matthew, Z., Rob, F.: Visualizing and understanding convolutional networks. In: European Conference on Computer Vision, pp. 818–833 (2014)

14. Oquab, M., Bottou, L., Laptev, I., Sivic, J.: Learning and transferring mid-level image representations using convolutional neural networks. In: IEEE Conference on Computer Vision and Pattern Recognition, pp. 1717–1724 (2014)

15. Krizhevsky, A., Sutskever, I., Hinton, G.E.: Imagenet classification with deep convolutional neural networks. Adv. Neural Inf. Process. Syst. **25**, 1097–1105 (2012)

16. Winder, S., Hua, G., Brown, M.: Picking the best daisy. In: IEEE Computer Vision and Pattern Recognition, pp. 178–185 (2009)

17. Manivannan, S., Li, W., Akbar, S., Wang, R., Zhang, J., McKenna, S.J.: An automated pattern recognition system for classifying indirect immunofluorescence images of HEp-2 cells and specimens. Pattern Recogn. **51**, 12–26 (2016)

18. Manivannan, S., Li, W., Akbar, S., Wang, R., Zhang, J., McKenna, S.J.: HEp-2 cell classification using multi-resolution local patterns and ensemble SVMs. In: I3A 1st workshop on Pattern Recognition Techniques for Indirect Immunoflurescence Images, in International Conference on Pattern Recognition (2014)

19. Boiman, O., Shechtman, E., Irani, M.: In defense of nearest-neighbor based image classification. In: IEEE Computer Vision and Pattern Recognition, pp. 1–8 (2008)

20. Zhen, X., Shao, L., Zheng, F.: Discriminative embedding via image-to-class distances. In: British Machine Vision Conference (2014)

21. Wang, Z., Hu, Y., Chia, L.T.: Image-to-class distance metric learning for image classification. In: European Conference on Computer Vision, pp. 706–719 (2010)

22. Bingham, E., Mannila, H.: Random projection in dimensionality reduction: applications to image and text data. In: ACM Knowledge Discovery and Data Mining, pp. 245–250 (2001)
23. Wang, J., Yang, J., Yu, K., Lv, F., Huang, T., Gong, Y.: Locality-constrained linear coding for image classification. In: IEEE Computer Vision and Pattern Recognition, pp. 3360–3367 (2010)
24. Chang, C.C., Lin, C.J.: LIBSVM: a library for support vector machines. ACM Trans. Intell. Syst. Technol. **2**, 27:1–27:27 (2011)
25. Engelhardt, S., Ameling, S., Paulus, D., Wirth, S.: Features for classification of polyps in colonoscopy. In: CEUR Workshop Proceedings (2010)
26. Maroulis, D.E., Iakovidis, D.K., Karkanis, S.A., Karras, D.A.: CoLD: a versatile detection system for colorectal lesions in endoscopy video-frames. Comput. Methods Programs Biomed. **70**, 151–166 (2003)
27. Li, W., Manivannan, S., Zhang, J., Trucco, E., McKenna, S.J.: Gland segmentation in colon histology images using hand-crafted features and convolutional neural networks. In: IEEE International Symposium on Biomedical Imaging (2016)
28. Jia, Y., Shelhamer, E., Donahue, J., Karayev, S., Long, J., Girshick, R., Guadarrama, S., Darrell, T.: Caffe: convolutional architecture for fast feature embedding. arXiv preprint arXiv:1408.5093 (2014)

Evaluation of i-Scan Virtual Chromoendoscopy and Traditional Chromoendoscopy for the Automated Diagnosis of Colonic Polyps

Georg Wimmer[1]([⊠]), Michael Gadermayr[2], Roland Kwitt[1], Michael Häfner[3], Dorit Merhof[2], and Andreas Uhl[1]

[1] Department of Computer Sciences, University of Salzburg, Salzburg, Austria
gwimmer@cosy.sbg.ac.at
[2] Interdisciplinary Imaging and Vision Institute Aachen,
RWTH Aachen University, Aachen, Germany
[3] St. Elisabeth Hospital, Vienna, Austria

Abstract. Image enhancement technologies, such as chromoendoscopy and digital chromoendoscopy were reported to facilitate the detection and diagnosis of colonic polyps during endoscopic sessions. Here, we investigate the impact of enhanced imaging technologies on the classification accuracy of computer-aided diagnosis systems. Specifically, we determine if image representations obtained from different imaging modalities are significantly different and experimentation is performed to figure out the impact of utilizing differing imaging modalities in the training and validation sets. Finally, we examine if merging the images of similar imaging modalities for training the classification model can be effectively applied to improve the accuracy.

Keywords: Colonic polyps · Endoscopy · Imaging modalities · i-Scan · Chromoendoscopy · Automated diagnosis

1 Introduction

Image enhancement technologies, such as chromoendoscopy and digital chromoendoscopy (such as narrow band imaging (NBI), Pentax's i-Scan or Fujinon's FICE), have become largely available in daily practice. These technologies apply different strategies to facilitate detection and histological prediction of colonic polyps compared to traditional white-light (WL) endoscopy and can be subdivided into conventional chromoendoscopy and digital chromoendoscopy:

1. Conventional chromoendoscopy (CC) came into clinical use 40 years ago. Staining the mucosa using (indigocarmine) dye spray enables an easier detection and classification of colonic polyps.

G. Wimmer, M. Gadermayr—Equal contributions.

© Springer International Publishing AG 2017
T. Peters et al. (Eds.): CARE 2016, LNCS 10170, pp. 59–71, 2017.
DOI: 10.1007/978-3-319-54057-3_6

2. Digital chromoendoscopy is a technique to facilitate "chromoendoscopy without dyes" [18] and can be subdivided in optical (NBI) and virtual chromoendoscopy (FICE, iScan):
   – Optical chromoendoscopy: In NBI, narrow bandpass filters are placed in front of a conventional white-light source to enhance the detail of certain aspects of the surface of the mucosa.
   – Virtual chromoendoscopy: The i-Scan (Pentax) image processing technology [20] is a digital contrast method which consists of combinations of surface enhancement, contrast enhancement and tone enhancement. i-Scan 1 performs surface enhancement augmenting pit patterns and surface details, providing assistance to the detection of dysplastic areas. This mode enhances light-to-dark contrast by obtaining luminance intensity data for each pixel and adjusting it to accentuate mucosal surfaces. i-Scan 2 expands on i-Scan 1 and additionally performs tone enhancement. It assists by intensifying boundaries, margins, surface architecture and difficult-to-discern polyps. i-Scan 3 is similar to i-Scan 2 with increased illumination and emphasis on the visualization of vascular features. This mode focuses on accentuating the vascular architecture.

   The FICE system (Fujinon) decomposes images by wavelength and then directly reconstructs images with enhanced mucosal surface contrast.

   Both systems (i-Scan and FICE) apply post-processing to the reflected light.

   In this work, we are primarily interested in traditional WL endoscopy, the i-Scan technology and chromoendoscopy, as imaging modalities (all using high definition (HD) endoscopes). Clinical studies about the effectiveness of these image enhancement technologies for the detection and classification of colonic polyps came to the following conclusions: In [16], it was shown that in case of HD endoscopes, chromoendoscopy and i-Scan are better suited for the detection and prediction of neoplastic lesions than traditional WL endoscopy. In [1], the prediction rates for small colonic polyps were compared using HD endoscopy, once again using either WL endoscopy, chromoendoscopy or the i-Scan technology. In this study, no significant differences were found between the results of the three imaging technologies. In [2], NBI, i-Scan and WL endoscopy were used for the histological prediction of diminutive colonic polyps, once again using HD endoscopes. In this study, NBI and i-Scan showed distinctly higher results than WL endoscopy. Outcomes with NBI and i-Scan were similar. All of these three studies reported higher results in case of the i-Scan technology compared to traditional WL endoscopy, although in one of the studies no significant difference was found. Based on these studies, the i-Scan technology can be considered as equivalent to NBI and chromoendoscopy when HD endoscopes are used. In [2,27], HD endoscopy combined with i-Scan was compared with standard (low definition) WL endoscopy. It was found that HD endoscopy in combination with i-Scan achieves significantly higher detection rates compared to standard WL endoscopy.

Previous works on the computer assisted diagnosis of colonic polyps based on highly detailed images can be divided in three categories, depending on the used endoscopes and imaging modalities:

1. High definition endoscopy combined with the i-Scan technology and with or without staining the mucosa [8,11]
2. High-magnification endoscopy combined with NBI [7,26]
3. High-magnification chromoendoscopy [10,13].

1.1 Contribution

In this work, we compare the prediction rates utilizing traditional WL endoscopy, chromoendoscopy, i-Scan and combinations of these imaging modalities. In contrast to previous works about the impact of different imaging modalities, automated diagnosis systems are deployed for the classification of the polyps instead of a manual classification performed by endoscopists. The authors of previous work on classifying colonic polyps based on HD-endoscopy in combination with WL endoscopy, chromoendoscopy and i-Scan came to the conclusion that chromoendoscopy complicates the differentiation of colonic polyps whereas i-Scan rather facilitates the differentiation of polyps [8,11]. Compared to these previous literature, our study is based on a distinctly larger number of different feature extraction methods, where each of these methods has already proven to be suited for the classification of colonic polyps in literature.

This study should answer three questions:

– Q1: Do the image representations differ between different modalities? This is first theoretically answered by applying a statistical test and then practical implications are considered by performing classifier training and evaluation based on different modalities.
– Q2: Should samples (from similar modalities) be collected for classifier training to obtain a larger training corpus exhibiting larger variability? Whereas Q1 is mainly of theoretical interest, Q2 should provide practically relevant outcomes.
– Q3: Which imaging modalities are best suited for the automated classification of colonic polyps.

2   Colonic Polyps Classification

Colonic polyps constitute a frequent finding and are known to either develop into cancer or to be precursors of colon cancer. Hence, an early assessment of the malignant potential of such polyps is important as this can lower the mortality rate drastically. As a consequence, a regular colon examination is recommended, especially for people at an age of 50 years and above. The current gold standard for the examination of the colon is colonoscopy. Modern endoscopic devices are able to take digital pictures or videos from inside the colon, allowing for a computer-assisted analysis with the goal of detecting and diagnosing abnormalities.

Colonic polyps are categorized into hyperplastic, adenomatous and malignant polyps. To determine a diagnosis based on the visual appearance of colonic polyps, the pit pattern classification scheme was proposed [22]. A pit is an opening of a colorectal crypt and the shape of a pit is denoted as pit pattern. The pit pattern classification scheme differentiates between six types. Type I (normal mucosa) and II (hyperplastic polyps) are characteristics of non-neoplastic lesions, type III-S, III-L and IV are typical for adenomatous polyps and type V is strongly suggestive to malignant cancer. Schemes and exemplar (zoom-endoscopic) images of the pit pattern types are presented in Fig. 1.

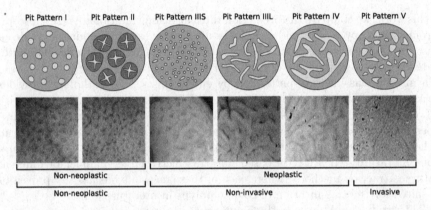

Fig. 1. The six pit pattern types along with exemplar images and their assigned classes in case of a two class (non-neoplastic vs neoplastic) and three class (non-neoplastic vs non-invasive vs invasive) differentiation

This classification scheme allows to differentiate between normal mucosa and hyperplastic lesions, adenomas (a pre-malignant condition), and malignant cancer based on the visual pattern of the mucosal surface. The removal of hyperplastic polyps is unnecessary and the removal of malignant polyps may be hazardous. Thus, the three-class scheme is useful to decide which lesions need not, which should, and which most likely must not be removed endoscopically. For these reasons, assessing the malignant potential of lesions at the time of colonoscopy is important, as this would allow to perform targeted biopsy. Apart from the three-classes case, the two-class classification scheme differentiating between non-neoplastic (pit pattern I and II) and neoplastic lesions (pit pattern III-V) is quite relevant in clinical practice [17]. Since the number of images showing malignant cancer is limited, we are only able to consider the two-classes case and have to omit the three-classes case.

The highly detailed images utilized in this work are gathered with high definition (HD) endoscopes based on traditional WL endoscopy, the i-Scan technology, chromoendoscopy as well as combinations of these image enhancement technologies.

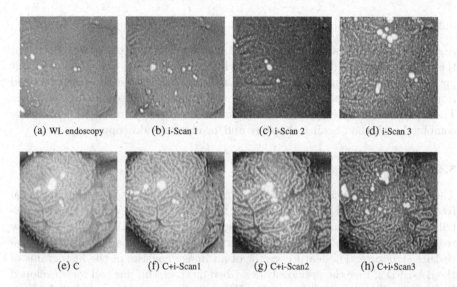

(a) WL endoscopy   (b) i-Scan 1   (c) i-Scan 2   (d) i-Scan 3

(e) C   (f) C+i-Scan1   (g) C+i-Scan2   (h) C+i-Scan3

Fig. 2. Images of a polyp using i-Scan and/or conventional chromoendoscopy (C)

In Fig. 2 images of an adenomatous polyp are shown, captured with eight different combinations of imaging modalities. Figure 2(a) shows the polyp using traditional WL endoscopy, (b,c,d) in combination with different i-Scan modes, (e) with chromoendoscopy and (f,g,h) with combinations of chromoendoscopy and the i-Scan technology.

3   Feature Extraction Methods

In this section we briefly describe the ten feature extraction methods utilized to differentiate between non-neoplastic and neoplastic lesions. All ten methods have proven to be well suited for the diagnosis of colonic polyps in literature.

3.1   CNN [25]

For this method, a convolutional neural network (CNN) pre-trained on the ImageNet ILSVRC challenge data (http://www.image-net.org/challenges/LSVRC/ is used as a fixed feature extractor. As CNN we deploy the VGG-f net from [3]. The images are fed through the CNN and the outputs of the first fully connected layer are extracted as feature.

3.2   Delaunay [10]

The first step of this method is to detect pits in the image using a local binary patterns operator. Based on the detected pit candidates, a Delaunay triangularization is computed and the edge length of the resulting triangles is utilized for classification of the colonic polyps. This method was especially developed for the classification of polyps based on zoom-endoscopic imagery.

3.3   BlobShape [8]

A segmentation similar to the watershed transformation is deployed to segment the image in connected regions (blobs), which model the pits and peaks of the pit pattern structure. Three shape features and one contrast feature are extracted from the detected blobs and histograms are computed based on these features. This method was developed for the classification of polyps using HD endoscopy combined with the i-Scan technology and/or chromoendoscopy.

3.4   BALFD [12]

The blob-adapted local fractal dimension (BA-LFD) is derived from the local fractal dimension (LFD) [28], a feature analysing changes in the intensity distribution in expanding circle shaped regions. In the BA-LFD approach, these regions are elliptic and the shape and size of the regions is adapted to the local texture structure. The feature vector of an image consists of the histograms of the BA-LFD's. Like the previously described method, this method was developed for the classification of polyps using HD endoscopy combined with the i-Scan technology and/or chromoendoscopy.

3.5   BSAGLFD [14]

The blob shape adapted gradient LFD (BSAGLFD) approach combines the BALFD and the BlobShape approach and turned out to achieve distinctly higher classification rates for the classification of colonic polyps than its two components. The BALFD and the BlobShape approach are applied to the original image as well as to the gradient magnitude image and the concatenation of the resulting features (using different weight factors for the BA-LFD and the BlobShape features) gives the feature vector of the BSAGLFD approach.

3.6   DT-CWT-Weibull [23]

The dual-tree complex wavelet transform (DT-CWT [19]) is a multi-scale and multi-orientation wavelet transform. The DT-CWT is applied using four decomposition levels. The feature extraction step is based on fitting a two-parameter Weibull distribution to the coefficient magnitudes of the DT-CWT sub-bands. The concatenation of the extracted Weibull features from all subbands gives the final feature vector of an image. Extracting Weibull features from DT-CWT, Gabor wavelet transform or shearlet transform subbands turned out to be highly suited for the classification of colonic polyps in [29].

3.7   GWT-Weibull [29]

The Gabor wavelet transform [24] is a multi-scale and multi-orientation wavelet transform. As for the DT-CWT, four decomposition levels are used and the subbands are fitted using the two-parameter Weibull distribution.

3.8   Shearlet-Weibull [29]

The shearlet transform [4] is based on the wavelet theory, but it offers more directional selectivity than wavelet transforms and a higher flexibility. The shearlet transform is applied using four decomposition levels with eight directions per decomposition level resulting in 32 subbands. Like for the two wavelet approaches, the final feature vector consists of the Weibull parameters extracted from the subbands.

3.9   LCVP [9]

Multi-scale local color vector patterns (LCVP) is based on local binary patterns (LBP). Whereas the LBP operator is applied to each color channel separately, LCVP constructs a color vector field from an image. Based on this field, the LCVP operator computes the similarity between neighboring pixels. The resulting image descriptor is a compact 1D-histogram. This method was especially developed for the classification of polyps using zoom-endoscopic imagery using chromoendoscopy.

3.10   VesselFeature [7]

In this approach, the blood vessel structure on polyps is segmented by means of the phase symmetry [21]. Eight features are computed describing the shape, the size, the contrast and the underlying color of the segmented vessels. This method is especially designed to analyze the vessel structures of polyps in NBI images and is potentially not suited for imaging modalities that are not designed to highlight the blood vessel structure.

4   Experimental Setup and Results

4.1   Experimental Setup

The eight image databases are acquired by extracting patches of size 256×256 from frames of HD-endoscopic (Pentax HiLINE HD+ 90i Colonoscope) videos. Most of the videos contain sequences from each of the eight imaging modalities (with or without i-Scan and with or without staining) but in some of the videos only a subset of the eight imaging modalities occur. Table 1 lists the number of images and patients per class for the eight databases, where each of the eight image databases is acquired under different imaging modalities. The patches utilized for our experiments are extracted from regions exhibiting histological findings.

Classification is performed utilizing leave-one-patient-out (LOPO) cross validation and a linear support vector machine classifier [5]. Compared to leave-one-out cross validation, the samples of one patient are either all in the training or all in the evaluation set to avoid any bias [15].

Table 1. Number of image patches and patients per class with and without staining the mucosa and with different i-Scan modes respectively with WL endoscopy (¬i-Scan)

i-Scan mode	No staining				Staining			
	¬i-Scan	i-Scan 1	i-Scan 2	i-Scan 3	¬i-Scan	i-Scan 1	i-Scan 2	i-Scan 3
Non − neoplastic								
Number of images	47	33	25	39	66	69	39	39
Number of patients	25	24	18	24	34	38	28	24
Neoplastic								
Number of images	86	88	80	80	85	85	74	63
Number of patients	66	66	64	63	66	65	62	55
Total no. of images	133	121	105	119	151	154	113	102

To investigate the similarity between the eight imaging modalities, each of the eight databases is classified using each of the eight databases for classifier training (always following the LOPO protocol). Thereby, for each feature extraction technique, 64 combinations (8 × 8) for training and evaluation are investigated and reported.

The motivation of this approach is to find out which imaging modalities are similar with respect to the outputs of the feature extraction methods and thereby can be potentially effectively combined.

Additionally we want to find out if it is better to use only those images for training that are from the same imaging modality as the considered evaluation image (to avoid differences between the training and validation samples) or if it is better to additionally utilize training images from other imaging modalities too, to increase the number of training samples.

To answer which groups of imaging modalities should be utilized for training, we additionally conduct three experiments using:

1. the images of the four databases without stained mucosa as training samples,
2. the images of the four databases with stained mucosa as training samples,
3. the images of all eight databases as training samples.

Again, LOPO is applied for these experiments and each of the eight image databases is classified using these three different training sets. To avoid any bias due to unbalanced evaluation data sets (especially the unequal number of images per class), we report the balanced classification accuracies only, equally weighting the sensitivity and the specificity.

To assess whether the distributions of the extracted features from the 10 feature extraction methods show statistically significant differences under different modalities (Q1), we conduct a series of two-sample hypothesis tests. In particular, we test for equality in feature distribution (i.e., the null-hypothesis). This is realized with the kernel-based two-sample test of Gretton et al. [6], using a standard RBF kernel (bandwidth parameter set to the median Euclidean distance between all samples) and 5000 permutations. For each pair of modalities, we tested all feature distributions and eventually computed the median over the resulting p-values of the 10 methods.

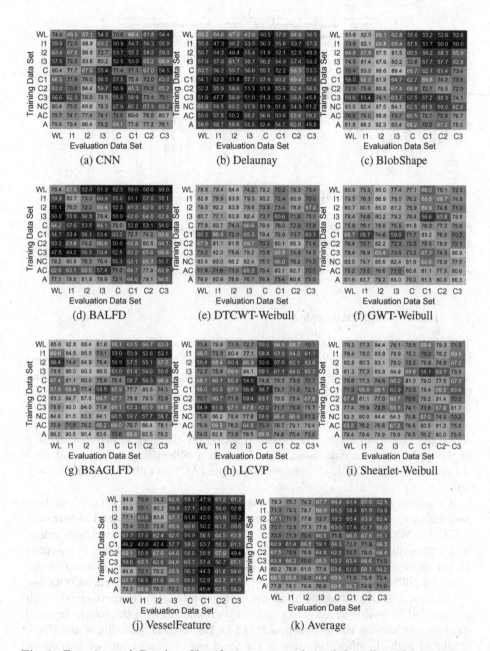

Fig. 3. Experimental Results: Classification was performed for all combinations of modalities (WL, I1, I2, I3, C, C1, C2, C3) for training and evaluation, where I1, I2, I3 denote the three i-Scan modes, C denotes chromoendoscopy and C1, C2, C3 denote chromoendoscopy in combination with the three i-Scan modes. Training was additionally conducted with all non-chromoscopic data (NC), all chromoscopic data (AC) and all eight data sets (A)

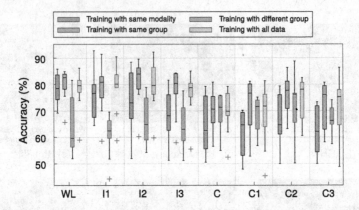

Fig. 4. Boxplot showing the distribution (median, quantiles, outliers) of accuracies above all image representations and training with: the same modality (red), the same modality-group (non-chromoscopy or chromoscopy, green), the different modality-group (blue) and all available data (yellow) (Color figure online)

4.2   Results and Discussion

The two-sample hypothesis tests showed that only the combinations (C+i-Scan2, C+i-Scan3) as well as (i-Scan2, C+i-Scan1) and (i-Scan2,C+i-Scan 2) showed no statistically significant difference at the 0.05 significance level. So the distributions of the extracted features are in general significantly different under different modalities.

In Fig. 3 we present the classification accuracies of the ten image representations. Each database was classified based on classifier training with each of the eight different databases, as well as on a collection containing all non-chromoendoscopic (NC), all chromoendoscopic (AC) and all (A) available data sets.

Considering the different image representations, we notice that the best performances on average were obtained with the wavelet based descriptors (DTCWT-Weibull, GWT-Weibull and Shearlet-Weibull). These methods exhibited a high discriminative power not only if training and evaluation is executed on the same modality (diagonal lines in Fig. 3), but also in the model transfer scenarios (different training and evaluation modalities). The accuracies obtained in the ideal scenario (diagonal lines) are partly even slightly outperformed which is supposed to be due to random effects in combination with the relatively small data sets. Other descriptors, such as BALFD, BSAGLFD, BlobShape and CNN, exhibited high classification rates in the ideal case (training and evaluation on the same data set) whereas rates mostly dropped distinctly for differing training and evaluation modalities. The VesselFeature method generally produced good outcomes only in combination with specific modalities. The performance of the Delaunay method was generally weak. In summary, regarding the performances of the ten image representations, we notice completely different behaviors with respect to varying classification scenarios.

Increasing the number of training samples by collecting additional data from other imaging modalities was partly effective. Especially WL endoscopy, i-Scan1 and i-Scan2 profited on average if all non-chromoscopic data was utilized for classifier training. The average accuracies (Fig. 3 (k)) improved from 78.3% to 80.2% (WL), from 74.2% to 78.8% (i-Scan1) and from 77.6% to 81.0% (i-Scan2), respectively. Interestingly, using the images of all imaging modalities as training samples did not further improve the averaged classification rates (except for i-Scan1). Considering the results of the chromoscopic evaluation sets, adding training samples of other chromoscopic image databases in general slightly decreases the averaged classification rates. Additionally adding non-chromoscopic image databases furtherly decreases the averaged classification rates. In general, the averaged classification rates are clearly higher for the evaluation sets without chromoendoscopy.

So additionally utilizing training samples of databases captured with the same chromoscopy mode (as the evaluation database) improves in four of eight cases the averaged classification rates. The results of utilizing training samples of all eight databases are in six of eight cases worse than these using only training samples of the same chromoscopy mode. Hence it can be assumed that especially the domain change between non-chromoscopy and chromoscopy image data is too pronounced to improve classification accuracy. The positive effect of more (diverse) training data is obviously vanished due to a distinctly changed feature distribution.

This behavior can be easier observed in Fig. 4, where the averaged accuracies over all image representations applying different training configurations are presented. Whereas training with the same group (non-chromoscopy or chromoscopy) led to improvements compared to training with the same imaging modality, the utilization of all data did not improve the outcome further. Training with the other group was always disadvantageous.

Based on these experiments, a clear statement on the overall best imaging modality cannot be made due to variably large training data sets. However, due to a consistent trend, we conclude that the highest distinctiveness is obtained without chromoendoscopy.

5   Conclusion

Our Experiments showed that feature distributions between different modalities are generally significantly different. For varying training and evaluation modalities, the obtained loss of accuracy strongly depended on the deployed feature extraction method. Especially wavelet-based image representations proved to be highly robust whereas others were less stable. For the wavelet-based methods, a combination of similar data for training (chromoscopy or non-chromoscopy samples) led to improved classification outcomes compared to using only training samples obtained with the same imaging modality. Considering the averaged accuracies over all methods, utilizing training samples of the same chromoscopic mode generally improves the results. The utilization of all available training data, did not perform equally well, which is supposed to be due to too distinct changes in image characteristics.

References

1. Basford, P., Longcroft, G., Bhandari, P.: Pwe-186 iscan in the evaluation of small colonic polyps: outcomes, learning curve from a large prospective series. Gut **61**(2), A372 (2012)
2. Bouwens, M., de Ridder, R., Masclee, A., Driessen, A., Riedl, R., Winkens, B., Sanduleanu, S.: Optical diagnosis of colorectal polyps using high-definition i-scan: an educational experience. World J. Gastroenterol. **19**(27), 4334–4343 (2013)
3. Chatfield, K., Simonyan, K., Vedaldi, A., Zisserman, A.: Return of the devil in the details: delving deep into convolutional nets. In: British Machine Vision Conference, BMVC 2014, Nottingham, UK, 1–5 September 2014
4. Easley, G., Labate, D., Lim, W.Q.: Sparse directional image representations using the discrete shearlet transform. Appl. Comput. Harmonic Anal. **25**(1), 25–46 (2008)
5. Fan, R.E., Chang, K.W., Hsieh, C.J., Wang, X.R., Lin, C.J.: LIBLINEAR: a library for large linear classification. J. Mach. Learn. Res. **9**, 1871–1874 (2008)
6. Gretton, A., Borgwardt, K., Rasch, M., Schölkopf, B., Smola, A.: A kernel two-sample test. JMLR **13**, 723–773 (2012)
7. Gross, S., Palm, S., Tischendorf, J.J.W., Behrens, A., Trautwein, C., Aach, T.: Automated classification of colon polyps in endoscopic image data. In: SPIE Proceedings, vol. 8315, pp. 83150W–83150W-8 (2012)
8. Häfner, M., Uhl, A., Wimmer, G.: A novel shape feature descriptor for the classification of polyps in HD colonoscopy. In: Menze, B., Langs, G., Montillo, A., Kelm, M., Müller, H., Tu, Z. (eds.) MCV 2013. LNCS, vol. 8331, pp. 205–213. Springer, Heidelberg (2014). doi:10.1007/978-3-319-05530-5_20
9. Häfner, M., Liedlgruber, M., Uhl, A., Vécsei, A., Wrba, F.: Color treatment in endoscopic image classification using multi-scale local color vector patterns. Med. Image Anal. **16**(1), 75–86 (2012)
10. Häfner, M., Liedlgruber, M., Uhl, A., Vécsei, A., Wrba, F.: Delaunay triangulation-based pit density estimation for the classification of polyps in high-magnification chromo-colonoscopy. Comput. Methods Programs Biomed. **107**(3), 565–581 (2012)
11. Häfner, M., Uhl, A., Wimmer, G.: Shape and size adapted local fractal dimension for the classification of polyps in HD colonoscopy. In: Proceedings of the IEEE International Conference on Image Processing 2014 (ICIP 2014), pp. 2299–2303, October 2014
12. Häfner, M., Uhl, A., Wimmer, G.: Shape and size adapted local fractal dimension for the classification of polyps in HD colonoscopy. In: Proceedings of the IEEE International Conference on Image Processing 2014 (ICIP 2014), October 2014
13. Häfner, M., Kwitt, R., Uhl, A., Gangl, A., Wrba, F., Vecsei, A.: Feature extraction from multi-directional multi-resolution image transformations for the classification of zoom-endoscopy images. Pattern Anal. Appl. **12**(4), 407–413 (2009)
14. Häfner, M., Tamaki, T., Tanaka, S., Uhl, A., Wimmer, G., Yoshida, S.: Local fractal dimension based approaches for colonic polyp classification. Med. Image Anal. **26**, 92–107 (2015)
15. Hegenbart, S., Uhl, A., Vécsei, A.: Survey on computer aided decision support for diagnosis of celiac disease. Comput. Biol. Med. **65**, 348–358 (2015)

16. Hoffman, A., Kagel, C., Goetz, M., Tresch, A., Mudter, J., Biesterfeld, S., Galle, P., Neurath, M., Kiesslich, R.: Recognition and characterization of small colonic neoplasia with high-definition colonoscopy using i-scan is as precise as chromoendoscopy. Dig. Liver Dis. **42**(1), 45–50 (2010)

17. Kato, S., Fu, K.I., Sano, Y., Fujii, T., Saito, Y., Matsuda, T., Koba, I., Yoshida, S., Fujimori, T.: Magnifying colonoscopy as a non-biopsy technique for differential diagnosis of non-neoplastic and neoplastic lesions. World J. Gastroenterol. **12**(9), 1416–1420 (2006)

18. Kiesslich, R.: Advanced imaging in endoscopy. Eur. Gastroenterol. Hepatol. Rev. **5**(1), 22–25 (2009)

19. Kingsbury, N.G.: The dual-tree complex wavelet transform: a new technique for shift invariance and directional filters. In: Proceedings of the IEEE Digital Signal Processing Workshop, DSP 1998, pp. 9–12. Bryce Canyon, USA, August 1998

20. Kodashima, S., Fujishiro, M.: Novel image-enhanced endoscopy with i-scan technology. World J. Gastroenterol. **16**(9), 1043–1049 (2010)

21. Kovesi, P.D.: Image features from phase congruency. Videre. J. Comput. Vision. Res. **1**(3), 2–26 (1999)

22. Kudo, S.E., Hirota, S., Nakajima, T., Hosobe, S., Kusaka, H., Kobayashi, T., Himori, M., Yagyuu, A.: Colorectal tumours and pit pattern. J. Clin. Pathol. **47**, 880–885 (1994)

23. Kwitt, R., Uhl, A.: Modeling the marginal distributions of complex wavelet coefficient magnitudes for the classification of zoom-endoscopy images. In: Proceedings of the IEEE Computer Society Workshop on Mathematical Methods in Biomedical Image Analysis (MMBIA 2007), Rio de Janeiro, Brasil, pp. 1–8 (2007)

24. Manjunath, B.S., Ma, W.Y.: Texture features for browsing and retrieval of image data. IEEE Trans. Pattern Anal. Mach. Intell. **18**(8), 837–842 (1996)

25. Razavian, A.S., Azizpour, H., Sullivan, J., Carlsson, S.: Cnn features off-the-shelf: an astounding baseline for recognition. In: Proceedings of the 2014 IEEE Conference on Computer Vision and Pattern Recognition Workshops, CVPRW 2014, pp. 512–519 (2014)

26. Tamaki, T., Yoshimuta, J., Kawakami, M., Raytchev, B., Kaneda, K., Yoshida, S., Takemura, Y., Onji, K., Miyaki, R., Tanaka, S.: Computer-aided colorectal tumor classification in NBI endoscopy using local features. Med. Image Anal. **17**(1), 78–100 (2013)

27. Testoni, P., Notaristefano, C., Vailati, C., Leo, M.D., Viale, E.: High-definition colonoscopy with i-scan: better diagnosis for small polyps and flat adenomas. World J. Gastroenterol. **18**(37), 5231–5239 (2012)

28. Varma, M., Garg, R.: Locally invariant fractal features for statistical texture classification. In: Proceedings of the IEEE International Conference on Computer Vision, Rio de Janeiro, Brazil, pp. 1–8, October 2007

29. Wimmer, G., Tamaki, T., Tischendorf, J., Häfner, M., Tanaka, S., Yoshida, S., Uhl, A.: Directional wavelet based features for colonic polyp classification. Med. Image Anal. **31**, 16–36 (2016)

ORBSLAM-Based Endoscope Tracking and 3D Reconstruction

Nader Mahmoud[1,2(✉)], Iñigo Cirauqui[3], Alexandre Hostettler[1],
Christophe Doignon[2], Luc Soler[1], Jacques Marescaux[1], and J.M.M. Montiel[3]

[1] IRCAD (Institut de Recherche contre les Cancers de l'Appareil Digestif),
Strasbourg, France
nader-mahmoud.ali@etu.unistra.fr
[2] ICube (UMR 7357 CNRS), Université de Strasbourg, Strasbourg, France
[3] Instituto de Investigación en Ingeniería de Aragón (I3A),
Universidad de Zaragoza, Zaragoza, Spain
josemari@unizar.es

Abstract. We aim to track the endoscope location inside the surgical
scene and provide 3D reconstruction, in real-time, from the sole input
of the image sequence captured by the monocular endoscope. This information offers new possibilities for developing surgical navigation and
augmented reality applications. The main benefit of this approach is
the lack of extra tracking elements which can disturb the surgeon performance in the clinical routine. It is our first contribution to exploit
ORBSLAM, one of the best performing monocular SLAM algorithms, to
estimate both of the endoscope location, and 3D structure of the surgical scene. However, the reconstructed 3D map poorly describe textureless
soft organ surfaces such as liver. It is our second contribution to extend
ORBSLAM to be able to reconstruct a semi-dense map of soft organs.
Experimental results on in-vivo pigs, shows a robust endoscope tracking even with organs deformations and partial instrument occlusions. It
also shows the reconstruction density, and accuracy against ground truth
surface obtained from CT.

Keywords: Endoscope tracking and navigation · Visual SLAM ·
Augmented reality

1 Introduction

Minimally Invasive Surgery (MIS) practice has several drawbacks for the surgeon, such as, lack of depth perception, or poor localization within operating
field due to the limited field of view. The intra-operative 3D reconstruction of
surgical scene simultaneous to tracking endoscope position in real-time provides
key information for many MIS tasks. These tasks include surgical navigation
(in case of flexible endoscope), and Augmented Reality (AR) overlies of pre-
operative medical data in the endoscope live video stream.

© Springer International Publishing AG 2017
T. Peters et al. (Eds.): CARE 2016, LNCS 10170, pp. 72–83, 2017.
DOI: 10.1007/978-3-319-54057-3_7

Recently, computer vision based algorithms have attracted the attention, for their success in providing intra-operative reconstruction of the surgical scene, and the tracking of the stereo-endoscope position [1,2]. However, these methods are not adapted to the commonly used monocular endoscope. Structure from motion (SfM) methods have been proposed to deal with monocular endoscope [3,4]. However, SFM methods requires offline batch processing, what makes them not suitable for real-time applications. Therefore, in [4] a tracking sensor is attached to the endoscope to estimate its position.

VSLAM (Simultaneous Location And Mapping from Visual sensor) is a popular topic in robotics, which aims at simultaneously building a 3D map of unknown environment while keep track of camera location. VSLAM use in MIS has been researched by Mountney et al. [5], who applied and extended the Extended Kalman Filter SLAM (EKF-SLAM) framework from Davison [6] to MIS environment, but with stereo-endoscope. For periodic liver deformation, Mountney and Yang [7] proposed to learn the parameters of the periodic motion first, and then use it to improve the VSLAM estimation.

In [8], Klein and Murray proposed the Parallel Tracking and Mapping (PTAM) algorithm that represented a breakthrough in visual SLAM. Lin et al. [2] adapted PTAM to a stereo-endoscope in order to reconstruct a denser 3D map than those made by EKF-SLAM systems. Due to non-rigid deformation in surgical scenes, the use of only a monocular endoscope has proven challenging. Grasa et al. [9] provided experimental evidence of the feasibility of monocular EKF SLAM in medical scenes. In [10], they provided extensive validation on in-vivo human sequences proofing its ability to be used for hernia defect measurements in hernia repair surgery.

Following the venue open by PTAM, the ORBSLAM system [11] has been proposed recently, it has proven as a robust camera tracking and mapping estimator with remarkable camera relocation capabilities. Our first contribution is researching ORBSLAM performance within MIS environments. By only re-tuning the system, the endoscope location was robustly tracked and relocated successfully after tracking loss. However, it is at the expense of a low map density, mainly due to the lack of repeatability of the ORB features in some body structures such as the liver. It is also our contribution a new matching algorithm to densify the map and hence improve the estimated 3D map. In the experimental, section we provide qualitative evaluation of the performance in several in-vivo pig sequences, including respiration, and tools cluttering the endoscope field of view. We also provide a quantitative assessment that yields an accuracy in the range between 3 mm to 4.5 mm when the VSLAM map points are compared with respect to a ground truth surface from CT. Additionally, the tracked endoscope location has been exploited to provide support for augmented reality overlays of preoperative models onto the endoscope live video stream.

2   ORBSLAM Overview

ORBSLAM is based on keyframes and nonlinear optimization as proposed in PTAM. It includes the covisibility information in the form of a graph as proposed in [12], in addition to bag of binary words DBoW2 proposed in [13] for place recognition. For large scale mapping, scale aware loop closing [14] is used. The system uses ORB [15] for feature detection and description in all processes, what boots the performance in the place recognition and loop closure operations. A complete description of the algorithm can be found in [11]. For the sake of completeness, we summarize next the more relevant steps: tracking, mapping and relocation.

Tracking. This task tracks the endoscope location sequentially in every frame of the live video. The 3D locations of the map points are assumed to be available, each of them with a valid ORB binary descriptor. At the current frame, an initial guess for the endoscope position is estimated from the previous frame by means of a motion model, then the map points are reprojected to estimate its image in the current frame. The ORB descriptor of each map point is compared with those of all the features detected inside a search region surrounding the predicted point. The feature point in the image with the smallest Hamming distance is selected as the match, only if it is over a threshold. Then the pose of the frame is refined by Huber robustified non-linear optimization of the reprojection error for the matched points. After the optimization stage, the matches are segmented as inliers or outliers according to the Huber threshold. Map points rendering outlier matches consistently during initialization are considered non reliable and do not survive in the initialization process.

Mapping. To build the 3D map of the scene, the system selects a set of frames from the endoscope sequence. This selected frames are called keyframes. Benefiting from the matches provided by the tracking process, the system estimates matches across the keyframes. Once the matches are available, the 3D location for the map points and the 3D poses for the keyframes are computed by bundle adjustment (BA). The algorithm sequentially computes the matches and iteratively improves the map accuracy, in a thread that runs in parallel with the tracking thread, but at lower frequency. The BA minimizes total Huber robustified reprojection error with respect to the keyframe positions, $\mathbf{X}_{WC_i}$, and the 3D map point locations, $\mathbf{X}_{Wj}$:

$$\underset{\mathbf{X}_{Wj}, \mathbf{X}_{WC_i}}{\arg\min} \sum_{i,j} \rho\left(\|\mathbf{u}_{ij} - \mathrm{CamProj}(\mathbf{X}_{Wj}, \mathbf{X}_{WC_i})\|\right) \tag{1}$$

where $\mathbf{u}_{ij}$ is the matched observation of the j-th map point by the i-th keyframe. CamProj codes the projection function including perspective and radial distortion. ρ denotes the robust Huber influence function. As the endoscope explores new areas of the scene not imaged previously, new keyframes are added to the map. After adding a new keyframe, new matches with respect to the previous keyframes are found to initialize new map points.

Initially, map points and keyframes are initialized in excess, then in a second stage a demanding rigorous is applied to select the fittest to survive. The reasons for culling a map point are: (1) The point cannot be tracked and matched in the following frames. (2) The projection rays used to triangulate the point in 3D render low parallax. (3) The triangulated point produces excessive reprojection error over the keyframes where it is observed. This severe selection of points have proven essential for robust performance in endoscope sequences. The keyframes whose 90% of the map points have been detected in at least other three keyframes are removed from the map, in order to keep just the more informative ones.

Map points are initialized by detecting ORB features at different image scales to achieve both scale and rotation invariance. One of the strong points of the algorithm is that ORB features are used both for mapping, and for the place recognition. Place recognition combines a Bag of Words built from the ORB binary descriptors, with the covisibility graph that determines all the keyframes that are observing the same 3D scene region.

Endoscope relocation. Tacking can be lost because of occlusion, feature deletion due to fast endoscope motion, or failure to match enough map points. Therefore, the endoscope has to be located with respect to the map from scratch. Relocation is also known as the kidnapped camera situation. All the keyframes of the map are stored in a Bag of Binary Words indexed database to recover the more similar keyframes in response to a query image. More crucially, thanks to the covisibility graph, the set of keyframes observing the same area of the map can be also recovered. After tracking loss, the ORB detected in the image gathered by the endoscope are used to query the database to detect the set of keyframes that are observing the same scene area as the endoscope image. Additionally, the system also provides a set of putative ORB matches between the image and a set of 3D points in the map. Then endoscope position is estimated by P3P and RANSAC. Once a valid endoscope pose is estimated, the tracking can be resumed.

3   Extending the Map Density

The mapping thread is responsible for creation/deletion of map points, and map refinement through BA. After new keyframe arrival, all of its ORB features are matched against closest keyframes, and all matched ORB points are triangulated and appended to the map. However, map points cannot be initialized on soft organs like liver, because they can not be repetitively detected along several frames in the sequence. We extended this initialization process to a second stage. Firstly, all matched ORB points are triangulated. Secondly, a cross-correlation guided by epipolar geometry is used to find matches for all unmatched ORB points in the newly added keyframe, according to Algorithm 1.

Figure 1 shows the map obtained by Algorithm 1. The original map created by ORBSLAM and its reprojection onto one liver image are shown in Fig. 1(a). Blue rectangles in Fig. 1(b,d,e) are keyframes describing endoscope trajectory, camera position in current image is displayed in green. Red points are ORB map points. A semi-dense map is obtained by reconstructing points in a sparse regions in the image and represented as green points in Fig. 1(d,e). More points will be reconstructed when exploring new regions. In subsequent frames, the newly reconstructed points (by Algorithm 1) are tracked, firstly, by Lucas-Kanade optical flow. Secondly, for all untracked points a cross-correlation search guided by epipolar geometry is performed using patch around the point extracted in the keyframe used for its 3D triangulation in Algorithm 1.

> **foreach** *Newly added KF (KF_C)* **do**
> > Get 4 neighbors KFs with significant baseline
> > **foreach** *Neighbor KF (KF_N)* **do**
> > > **foreach** *unmatched ORB feature (P_c) in KF_C* **do**
> > > > - Extract a rectangular correlation patch
> > > > - Patch crosscorrelation around epipolar segment in KF_N
> > > > - Threshold on maximal distance to epipolar line
> > > > - Triangulate map point from matched two observations
> > > > - Remove points with negative depth relative to KF_C and KF_N
> > > > - Threshold on maximal reprojection error onto KF_C and KF_N
> > > > - Remove point if depth different from median depth in KF_C
> > >
> > > end
> >
> > end
>
> end

Algorithm 1. Cross-correlation search for 3D point triangulation

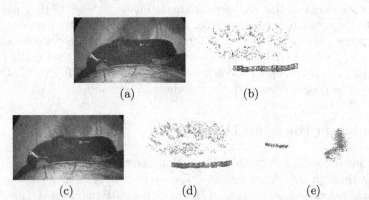

(a)   (b)

(c)   (d)   (e)

Fig. 1. Algorithm 1 semi-dense map. (a) Reprojection of the ORB points (yellow). (b) ORBSLAM 3D map. (c) Reprojection of Algorithm 1 map points. (d, e) Algorithm 1 map (green) and ORBSLAM map (red), from two different points of view (Color figure online)

4   Experimental Results

The performance was evaluated with several in-vivo pig laparoscopy sequences. The endoscope camera was calibrated following [16]. Next we detail the different experiments. More details can be appreciated in our video [17]

4.1 ORBSLAM Performance Evaluation

We re-tune the ORBSLAM to overcame the key factors limiting its performance when processing endoscope sequences, we report modifications relative to the ORBSLAM standard rigid case:

Search region in tracking. For tracking, map points are reprojected in the image, and each one of them defines a search region in which a match with an image keypoint is attempted. We have increased the size of the search region in a factor 1.5 (0.5 pixel), not to loose some matches due to potential deformation.

Parallax threshold at point initialization. When a map point is created, it is enforced to have at least a threshold parallax to ensure that its location in 3D is accurate. Minimum parallax is increased in a factor of 5, it becomes $1.4035°$, to increase the accuracy in the triangulated points.

Reprojection error threshold. A maximum threshold is allowed in the distance between the reprojected map point and the image keypoints used for its triangulation. We reduced this threshold in a factor 10, it becomes 0.5991, to ensure that only rigid scene points are included eventually in the map.

Hamming distance threshold. We reduce the allowed Hamming distance between descriptors of matched image points. We decreased it by a factor 0.9, it becomes 45 bit, to enforce more similarity in the accepted matches.

We have found that the endoscope tracking qualitatively quite robust and accurate. However, there are many areas of the scene where the system is unable to track map points, being able to match only 24% of the map points visible in the image. The main reason for this failure in matching, around 50% of the potential matches, is that ORB detector is not able to detect repeatable points on soft organs, such as liver. Also, BA in mapping process considers 11% of the map points as non-rigid, this percentage raises up to 25% in areas with visually high non-rigid component. Despite the low number of matched map points, the system was able to compute an sparse map. Figure 2(d) shows the reconstructed map which consisted of 66 keyframes and 1566 map points. In this part of the sequence the endoscope was fixed relative to the operating table, Fig. 2(e) and (f) show the ability to estimate the breathing motion, because of the pig breathing there was a forward-backward motion of the diaphragm able to be seen in the camera trajectory.

Additionally, the system was able to accurately relocate the endoscope location after tracking loss. In Fig. 3, after the exploration phase of the abdominal cavity, the endoscope was extracted outside the cavity while looking at the liver, and it is later reinserted imaging the spleen. Since, several spleen points had been mapped before, the system was able to relocate the endoscope location within 3 s.

Finally, the system has also been tested with challenging gastroscopy sequences which contains reflection and abrupt movements. It was able to track the endoscope location and reconstruct 3D map of the scene (cf. Fig. 4). The average tracking time per frame was approximately 25 ms on desktop PC with Intel(R) Core d −3337U CPU @ 1.80 GHz with 6 GB RAM.

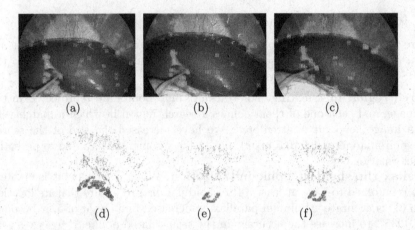

Fig. 2. ORBSLAM performance. (a–c) images with reprojected map points(green points). (d) Reconstructed map points (red) and keyframes (endoscope tip trajectory). (e–f) Breathing motion, current endoscope location is shown as a green rectangle. (e) and (f) during inhale and exhale, respectively. (Color figure online)

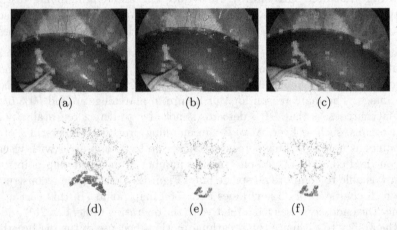

Fig. 3. Relocation ability. (a) Consecutive stages from left to right: successful tracking while observing the liver, tracking loss when endoscope was extracted, endoscope inserted again imaging the spleen, relocation. (b,c) The arrows refer to the endoscope locations before tracking lost, and after relocation

4.2   Estimation of Reconstruction Error

To evaluate the error associated with the reconstructed point cloud of the scene, two pigs were used inside computed tomography (CT) room to obtain in-vivo sequences with CT ground truth surface. A monocular endoscope explores the abdominal cavity before any interaction with the liver. Then a CT scan was performed while the endoscope was fixed by means of an articulated arm as shown in Fig. 5. In all CT acquisitions, the tip of the endoscope was included in

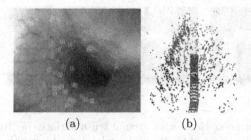

(a)   (b)

Fig. 4. Gastroscopy sequence. (a) Esophagus with tracked points. (b) Reconstructed map (red and black points), keyframes (blue rectangles) and current endoscope location (green rectangle). (Color figure online)

the CT, to be segmented and extracted from the CT images. The length of the recorded sequences ranged between 2 to 10 min.

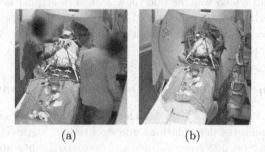

(a)   (b)

Fig. 5. Data acquisition. (a) Video recording. (b) CT acquisition while endoscope was fixed and its tip inside the abdominal cavity

The abdominal surface was segmented from CT images and considered as ground truth. In order to compare with the VSLAM map, firstly, the endoscope was segmented from CT images and its position w.r.t the surface was computed using [18]. Endoscope position estimated by ORBSLAM and by [18] were aligned, however VLSAM cannot recover the scene scale (λ), and [18] cannot recover the endoscope roll angle (θ) so additional scale and rotational alignment was needed before comparing the two scene maps. The alignment is not a critical process, brute-force search to find both the scale and the roll angle that minimize the distance between the VSLAM map and the CT surface was used.

The distance is defined as the euclidean distance between each point in the VSLAM map its closest one on the CT surface. The closest point on the surface is the one with smallest perpendicular distance. So the cost function for the Brute-force optimization is:

$$\underset{\lambda, R(\theta)}{\arg\min} \sqrt{\frac{1}{N} \sum_{i=1}^{N} ||P_i - \lambda \cdot R(\theta) \cdot Q_i||^2} \qquad (2)$$

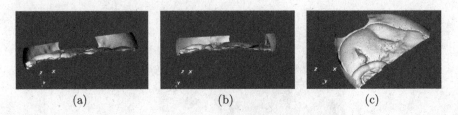

(a)   (b)   (c)

Fig. 6. Alignment of point cloud with ground truth surface. (a) Reconstructed ORB points. (b) and (c) alignment of ORB points and points obtained by Algorithm 1 from different directions. Red line is the estimated endoscope position by [18].

where P_i are CT surface points closest point and Q_i are the N VSLAM map points. λ and $R(\theta)$ are the scale factor and rotation matrix calculated from the roll angle, respectively. Only 80% of the points are considered in RMSE computation. The remaining 20% are either outliers or points reconstructed on the diaphragm wall which was outside the CT field of acquisition. The obtained RMSE of considering only reconstructed ORB points was approximately 3 mm (cf. Fig. 6(a)). The RMSE of the semi-dense map obtained by Algorithm 1 was approximately 4.1 mm (cf. Fig. 6(b–c)).

4.3 Evaluation with Instrument Occlusion and Deformations

Several pig liver sequences are used, which contains instruments interacting with the liver, what generates deformations and occlusions. Figure 7(b–d) shows the endoscope tracking on one liver sequence, where red points are reconstructed ORB points and green points are reconstructed by Algorithm 1. The estimated endoscope position in the current frame is represented in green rectangle, while the blue rectangles represent the trajectory described as past keyframe positions. Yellow and blue points in Fig. 7(a) are the reprojection of ORB points and points reconstructed by Algorithm 1, respectively. We use the same colors for all subsequent figures. As it can be noticed, more points were reconstructed particularly on the liver (Fig. 7(e)). The number of the recovered 3D map points were about 4599 with 58 keyframes.

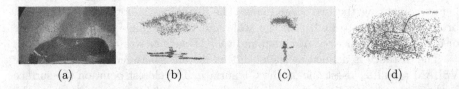

(a)   (b)   (c)   (d)

Fig. 7. Endoscope tracking and reconstructed 3D map from exploration phase. (a-c) Reconstructed points and keyframe positions from different directions. (e) Reconstructed points colored using the same RGB color of the 2D features (Color figure online)

Figure 8 shows results on different sequences including different deformations and partial scene occlusion due to an instrument. Figure 8(c) shows, from a top view, the endoscope position w.r.t the reconstructed 3D map. The reconstructed 3D map, keyframes and current endoscope position for Fig. 8(d) are displayed in Fig. 8(e,f). For first row sequence, the size of the reconstructed map were 6750 points, 3263 points for second row sequence and 3740 points for third row sequence.

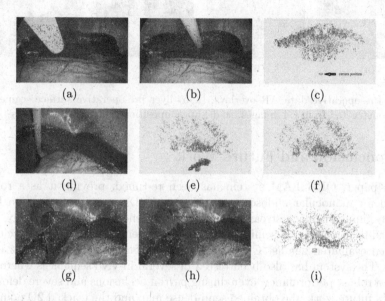

Fig. 8. Endoscope tracking and reconstructed 3D map during different deformations

It is worth noting that the liver of the second pig (cf. Fig. 8 second and third rows) was totally texture-less and it was hardly to detect features on its surface, but the system was able to reconstruct many points on liver. The endoscope location was successfully tracked during the interaction with liver in all sequences (cf. Fig. 8(b,d,g)). In case of tracking failure due to feature deletion during fast endoscope movements the system was able to relocate the endoscope location once the endoscope had moved and few ORB features were detected. Algorithm 1 is allocated in the tracking thread, increasing its computation time as shown in Table 1, which reports the average additional time due to the reconstruction and matching of all points.

The estimated endoscope location was used to superimpose AR onto one video sequence. The AR insertion was the liver pre-operative surface segmented from CT images in addition to hepatic veins. The pre-operative liver surface and hepatic veins were manually registered in first few frames, and then successfully tracked through out the whole video. Few frames are randomly picked to show the augmented results in Fig. 9.

Table 1. Average time (in ms) of different tasks

Mapping		Tracking		
New points triangulation	ORB triangulation	ORB matching	L-K opt. flow & cross corr	Tracking time
25.3	379.2	13.3	66.2	105.2

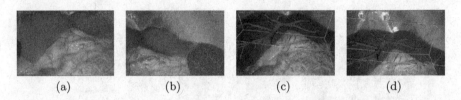

(a)	(b)	(c)	(d)

Fig. 9. Pre-operative data AR overlays. (a–b) liver pre-operative surface segmented and reconstructed from CT images. [c–d] superimposition of liver hepatic veins.

5   Conclusion and Future Work

In this paper, ORBSLAM system has been re-tuned, proving it as a robust method for monocular endoscope tracking and 3D scene reconstruction from the only input of image stream gathered by the endoscope. Additionally, it is extended to reconstruct a semi-dense map of the scene. The scene map accuracy has been evaluated against CT ground truth surface and achieving 3–4.1 mm RMSE. The system has also been tested in several in-vivo sequences where displayed a robust performance, even during partial occlusions and severe deformations. In future work, the obtained semi-dense map and the tracked 2D points in the image will be used to estimate the non-rigid organ deformations using shape from template techniques.

Ethical approval: All applicable international, national, and/or institutional guidelines for the care and use of animals were followed.

Acknowledgments. This work is supported by the Dirección General de Investigación Centífica y Técnica of Spain under Project RT-SLAM DPI2015-67275-P

References

1. Stoyanov, D., Scarzanella, M.V., Pratt, P., Yang, G.-Z.: Real-time stereo reconstruction in robotically assisted minimally invasive surgery. In: Jiang, T., Navab, N., Pluim, J.P.W., Viergever, M.A. (eds.) MICCAI 2010. LNCS, vol. 6361, pp. 275–282. Springer, Heidelberg (2010). doi:10.1007/978-3-642-15705-9_34
2. Lin, B., Johnson, A., Qian, X., Sanchez, J., Sun, Y.: Simultaneous tracking, 3D reconstruction and deforming point detection for stereoscope guided surgery. In: Liao, H., Linte, C.A., Masamune, K., Peters, T.M., Zheng, G. (eds.) AE-CAI/MIAR -2013. LNCS, vol. 8090, pp. 35–44. Springer, Heidelberg (2013). doi:10.1007/978-3-642-40843-4_5

3. Wu, C.-H., Sun, Y.-N., Chang, C.-C.: Three-dimensional modeling from endoscopic video using geometric constraints via feature positioning. IEEE Trans. Biomed. Eng. **54**(7), 1199–1211 (2007)

4. Sun, D., Liu, J., Linte, C.A., Duan, H., Robb, R.A.: Surface reconstruction from tracked endoscopic video using the structure from motion approach. In: Liao, H., Linte, C.A., Masamune, K., Peters, T.M., Zheng, G. (eds.) AE-CAI/MIAR -2013. LNCS, vol. 8090, pp. 127–135. Springer, Heidelberg (2013). doi:10.1007/ 978-3-642-40843-4_14

5. Mountney, P., Stoyanov, D., Davison, A., Yang, G.-Z.: Simultaneous stereoscope localization and soft-tissue mapping for minimal invasive surgery. In: Larsen, R., Nielsen, M., Sporring, J. (eds.) MICCAI 2006. LNCS, vol. 4190, pp. 347–354. Springer, Heidelberg (2006). doi:10.1007/11866565_43

6. Davison, A.J.: Real-time simultaneous localisation and mapping with a single camera. In: ICCV, pp. 1403–1410 (2003)

7. Mountney, P., Yang, G.-Z.: Motion compensated SLAM for image guided surgery. In: Jiang, T., Navab, N., Pluim, J.P.W., Viergever, M.A. (eds.) MIC-CAI 2010. LNCS, vol. 6362, pp. 496–504. Springer, Heidelberg (2010). doi:10.1007/ 978-3-642-15745-5_61

8. Klein, G., Murray, D.W.: Parallel tracking and mapping for smallar workspaces. In: ISMAR, pp. 225–234 (2007)

9. Grasa, O.G., Civera, J., Montiel, J.M.M.: EKF monocular SLAM 3D modeling, measuring and augmented reality from endoscope image sequences. In: MICCAI 2009, vol. 2 (2009)

10. Grasa, O.G., Bernal, E., Casado, S., Gil, I., Montiel, J.M.M.: Visual SLAM for hand-held monocular endoscope. IEEE Trans. Med. Imaging **33**(1), 135–146 (2014)

11. Mur-Artal, R., Montiel, J.M.M., Tardós, J.D.: ORB-SLAM: a versatile and accurate monocular SLAM system. IEEE Trans. Robot. **31**(5), 1147–1163 (2015)

12. Strasdat, H., Davison, A.J., Montiel, J.M.M., Konolige, K.: Double window optimization for constant time visual SLAM. In: IEEE International Conference on Computer Vision (ICCV), pp. 2352–2359 (2011)

13. Galvez-López, D., Tardós, J.D.: Bags of binary words for fast place recognition in image sequences. IEEE Trans. Robot. **28**(5), 1188–1197 (2012)

14. Strasdat, H., Montiel, J.M.M., Davison, A.J.: Scale drift-aware large scale monocular SLAM. In: Robotics: Science and Systems VI (2010)

15. Rublee, E., Rabaud, V., Konolige, K., Bradski, G.: ORB: an efficient alternative to SIFT or SURF. In: IEEE International Conference on Computer Visition (ICCV), pp. 2564–2571 (2011)

16. Zhang, Z.: A flexible new technique for camera calibration. IEEE Trans. Pattern Anal. Mach. Intell. **22**(11), 1330–1334 (2000)

17. Youtube. ORBSLAM-based Endoscope Tracking and 3D Reconstruction [Video file], 1 August 2016. https://www.youtube.com/watch?v=UzPjHQX5-9A. Accessed

18. Bernhardt, S., Nicolau, S.A., Agnus, V., Soler, L., doignon, C., Marescaux, J.: Automatic detection of endoscope in intraoperative CT image: application to AR guidance in laparoscopic surgery. IEEE 11th International Symposium on Biomedical Imaging (ISBI), pp. 563–567 (2014)

Real-Time Segmentation of Non-rigid Surgical Tools Based on Deep Learning and Tracking

Luis C. García-Peraza-Herrera[1(✉)], Wenqi Li[1], Caspar Gruijthuijsen[4],
Alain Devreker[4], George Attilakos[3], Jan Deprest[5],
Emmanuel Vander Poorten[4], Danail Stoyanov[2], Tom Vercauteren[1],
and Sébastien Ourselin[1]

[1] Translational Imaging Group, CMIC, University College London, London, UK
luis.herrera.14@ucl.ac.uk
[2] Surgical Robot Vision Group, CMIC, University College London, London, UK
[3] University College London Hospitals, London, UK
[4] Katholieke Universiteit Leuven, Leuven, Belgium
[5] Universitair Ziekenhuis Leuven, Leuven, Belgium

Abstract. Real-time tool segmentation is an essential component in computer-assisted surgical systems. We propose a novel real-time automatic method based on Fully Convolutional Networks (FCN) and optical flow tracking. Our method exploits the ability of deep neural networks to produce accurate segmentations of highly deformable parts along with the high speed of optical flow. Furthermore, the pre-trained FCN can be fine-tuned on a small amount of medical images without the need to hand-craft features. We validated our method using existing and new benchmark datasets, covering both *ex vivo* and *in vivo* real clinical cases where different surgical instruments are employed. Two versions of the method are presented, non-real-time and real-time. The former, using only deep learning, achieves a balanced accuracy of 89.6% on a real clinical dataset, outperforming the (non-real-time) state of the art by 3.8% points. The latter, a combination of deep learning with optical flow tracking, yields an average balanced accuracy of 78.2% across all the validated datasets.

1 Introduction

Tool detection, segmentation and tracking is a core technology that has many potential applications. It may for example be used to increase the context-awareness of surgeons in the operating room [1]. In the context of delicate surgical interventions, such as fetal [2] and ophthalmic surgery [3], providing the clinical operator with accurate real-time information about the surgical tools could be highly valuable and help to avoid human errors. Identifying tools is also part

Electronic supplementary material The online version of this chapter (doi:10.1007/978-3-319-54057-3_8) contains supplementary material, which is available to authorized users.

T. Peters et al. (Eds.): CARE 2016, LNCS 10170, pp. 84–95, 2017.
DOI: 10.1007/978-3-319-54057-3_8

of other computational pipelines such as mosaicking, visual servoing and skills assessment. Image mosaicking can provide reconstructions larger than the image provided by the usual endoscopic view. The mosaic is normally generated by stitching endoscopic images as the endoscope moves across the operating site [4]. However, surgical tools present in the images occlude the surgical scene being reconstructed. Real-time instrument detection and tracking facilitates the localisation of the instruments and the further separation from the underlying tissue, so that the final mosaic only contains patient's tissue. Another application of tool segmentation is visual servoing of articulated or flexible surgical robots. As the dexterity of the instruments rises [5], it becomes increasingly difficult for the surgeon to understand the shape of these instruments. With the miniaturisation of said instruments, the kinematics of these devices become less deterministic due to effects from friction, hysteresis and backlash alongside with increased instrument compliance and safety. Furthermore, it is challenging to embed position or shape sensing on them without increasing their size. A key advantage of visual tool tracking versus fiducial markers or auxiliary technologies is that there is no need to modify the current workflow or propose alternative exotic instruments. Previous work has addressed detection [6], localisation [7] and pose estimation of instruments [8] using different cues and classification strategies. For example, employing information about the geometry of the instruments [9], fiducial markers [10], 3D coordinates of the insertion point [11], fusing visual and kinematic information [12] and through multi-class pixel-wise classification of colour, texture and position features with different machine learning techniques such as Random Forests (RF) [7] and Boosted Decision Forests [1]. Recent advances in Region-based Convolutional Neural Networks (R-CNN) [13] and Region Proposal Networks (RPN) [14] have enabled the possibility of object detection (with a bounding box) near real-time (17 fps for images on Pascal VOC 2007 [15]). EndoNet [16] has been recently proposed as a solution for phase recognition and tool presence detection on laparoscopic videos. However, there is still a need for an automatically initialised real-time (i.e. camera frame rate) segmentation algorithm for non-rigid tools with unknown geometry and kinematics.

There are a number of challenges that need to be addressed for real-time detection and tracking of surgical instruments. Endoscopic images typically present a vast amount of specular reflections (from both tissue and instruments), which is a source of confusion for segmentation algorithms as pixels that look the same belong to different objects (e.g. background and foreground). Changing lighting conditions, shadows and motion blur, combined with the complexity of the scene and the motion of organs in the background are also a challenge, as can be observed in Fig. 1. As a result, anatomical structures and surgical instruments may look more similar than they actually are. Occlusions caused by body fluids and smoke also represent a major issue. Particularly for the case of fetal surgery, the turbidity of the amniotic fluid, makes the localisation of instruments really challenging, as can be observed in Fig. 1. Fetal surgery also has the additional difficulty of relying on miniature endoscopes that contain several tens of thousands of fibres in an imaging guide. Transformed into pixels the number of fibres

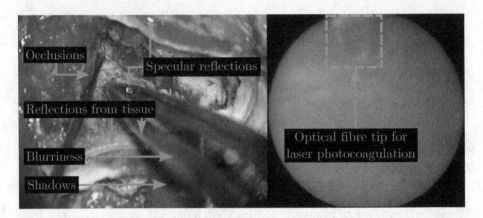

Fig. 1. Challenges encountered by tool detection and localisation algorithms in real interventions. *In vivo* neurosurgery [1] (left). Twin-to-twin transfusion syndrome laser photocoagulation (right).

results in a very poor resolution (e.g. 30 K in a KARL STORZ GMBH 11508 AAK curved fetoscope [17]).

To the best of our knowledge, in this paper, we present the first real-time ($\approx$30 fps) surgical tool segmentation pipeline. Our pipeline takes monocular video as input and produces a foreground/background segmentation based on both deep learning semantic labelling and optical flow tracking. The method is instrument-agnostic and can be used to segment different types of rigid or non-rigid instruments. We demonstrate that deep learning semantic labelling outperforms the state of the art on an open neurosurgical clinical dataset [1]. Our results also show competitive performance between real-time and non-real-time implementations of our method.

2   Methods

Convolutional-Neural-Network-based Segmentation. There are several benefits of using a Convolutional Neural Network (CNN) compared to other state-of-the-art machine learning approaches [1]. First, there is no need for trial and error to hand-craft features, as features are automatically extracted during the network training phase. As demonstrated in [18], automatic feature selection does not negatively affect the segmentation quality. Furthermore, CNNs can be pre-trained on large general purpose datasets from the Computer Vision community and fine-tuned with a small amount of domain-specific images, as explained in [19]. This particular feature of CNNs allows us to overcome the scarcity of labelled images faced by the CAI community. Therefore, it conveys the possibility of having an instrument segmentation mechanism that is not tool dependent, as demonstrated by our results.

Fully Convolutional Networks (FCN) are a particular type of CNN recently proposed by Long et al. [19]. As opposed to previous CNNs such as AlexNet [20] or VGG16 [21], FCN are tailored to perform semantic labelling rather than classification. However, the two are closely related as FCN are built from adapting and fine-tuning pre-trained classification networks. In order to achieve this conversion from classification to segmentation two key steps are performed. First, the fully connected (FC) layers of the classification network are replaced with convolutions so that spatial information is preserved. Second, *upsampling filters* (also called *deconvolution layers*) are employed to generate a multi-class pixel-level output segmentation that features the same size of the input image. An essential characteristic of the *upsampling filters* present in FCN is that their weights are not fixed, but initialised to perform bilinear interpolation and then learnt during the fine-tuning process. As a consequence, these networks are able to accept an arbitrary-sized input, produce a labelled output of equivalent dimensions and rely on end-to-end learning of labels and locations. That is, they behave as *deep non-linear filters* that perform semantic labelling. There are three versions of the FCN introduced by Long et al., FCN-8s (shown in Fig. 2), FCN-16s and FCN-32s (available in the CAFFE Model Zoo [22]). The difference between them being the use of intermediate outputs (such as the one coming from POOL_3 or POOL_4 in Fig. 2) in order to achieve finer segmentations.

In this work, we have adapted and fine-tuned the FCN-8s [19] for instrument segmentation. Its state-of-the-art performance in multi-class segmentation of general purpose computer vision datasets makes it a sensible choice for the task. The FCN-8s we employed was pre-trained on the PASCAL-context 59-class (60 including background) [23] dataset. As we are concerned with the separation of non-rigid surgical instruments from background, the structure of the network was adapted to provide only two scores per pixel by changing the number of outputs to just *two* in the scoring and upsampling layers. This modification of

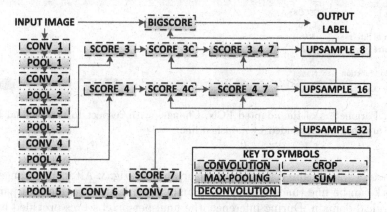

Fig. 2. Illustration of the FCN-8s network architecture, as proposed in [19]. In our method, the architecture of the network remains the same, but the number of outputs in SCORE_3, SCORE_4, SCORE_5, UPSAMPLE_8, UPSAMPLE_16 and UPSAMPLE_32 has been changed so that they produce only two scores per pixel, background and foreground.

Name	CONV_1_1	CONV_1_2	POOL_1	CONV_2_1	CONV_2_2	POOL_2
Type	Convolution	Convolution	Max-pooling	Convolution	Convolution	Max-pooling
Number of filters	64	64	N/A	128	128	N/A
Kernel size	3	3	2	3	3	2
Stride	1	1	2	1	1	2
Activation function	ReLU	ReLU	N/A	ReLU	ReLU	N/A

Name	CONV_3_1	CONV_3_2	CONV_3_3	POOL_3	CONV_4_1	CONV_4_2
Type	Convolution	Convolution	Convolution	Max-pooling	Convolution	Convolution
Number of filters	256	256	256	N/A	512	512
Kernel size	3	3	3	2	3	3
Stride	1	1	1	2	1	1
Activation function	ReLU	ReLU	ReLU	N/A	ReLU	ReLU

Name	CONV_4_3	POOL_4	CONV_5_1	CONV_5_2	CONV_5_3	POOL_5
Type	Convolution	Max-pooling	Convolution	Convolution	Convolution	Max-pooling
Number of filters	512	N/A	512	512	512	N/A
Kernel size	3	2	3	3	3	2
Stride	1	2	1	1	1	2
Activation function	ReLU	N/A	ReLU	ReLU	ReLU	N/A

Name	CONV_6	CONV_7	SCORE_3	SCORE_4	SCORE_7	UPSAMPLE_32
Type	Convolution	Convolution	Convolution	Convolution	Convolution	Deconvolution
Number of filters	4096	4096	2	2	2	2
Kernel size	7	1	1	1	1	4
Stride	1	1	1	1	1	2
Activation function	ReLU	ReLU	None	None	None	None

Name	UPSAMPLE_16	UPSAMPLE_8	SCORE_4_7	SCORE_3_4_7	SCORE_3C	SCORE_4C
Type	Deconvolution	Deconvolution	Sum	Sum	Crop	Crop
Number of filters	2	2	N/A	N/A	N/A	N/A
Kernel size	4	16	N/A	N/A	N/A	N/A
Stride	2	8	N/A	N/A	N/A	N/A
Activation function	None	None	None	None	None	None

Name	BIGSCORE
Type	Crop
Number of filters	N/A
Kernel size	N/A
Stride	N/A
Activation function	None

Fig. 3. Parameters of the adapted FCN. Changes with respect to the original FCN-8s [19] are shown surrounded by a dashed line.

parameters is highlighted within the dashed line in Fig. 3. After this change, the network can be fine-tuned with a small amount of data belonging to a particular surgical domain. During inference, the final per-pixel scores provided by the FCN are normalised and calculated via *argmax* to obtain per-pixel labels.

We have also implemented an improved learning process for the FCN. The optimiser selected to update the weights was the standard *Stochastic Gradient Descent* (SGD). A key hyper-parameter of the fine-tuning process is the *learning rate* (LR), which is the weight applied to the negative gradient used in the update rule of the optimisation. It has been recently shown in [24] that letting the learning rate fluctuate during the fine-tuning process achieves convergence to a higher accuracy in less number of iterations. This policy, introduced by Smith as Cyclical Learning Rate (CLR) [24], may be implemented with different shapes (e.g. triangular, parabolic, sinusoidal). However, all of them produce similar results in [24]. We therefore choose the triangular window for the sake of simplicity. As we are only interested in fine-tuning the network, the LR was constrained to a small value to tailor the parameters to the surgical domain without altering the behaviour of the network. In our case, the LR boundaries, momentum and weight decay were set to [1e-13, 1e-10], 0.99 and 0.0005, respectively.

Real-Time Segmentation Pipeline. The drawback of the FCN we used is that it cannot run in real-time. CAFFE performs forward evaluation in about 100 ms for a 500×500 RGB image using an NVIDIA GeForce GTX TITAN X GPU, but this computational time is well below the frame-rate of the endoscopic video, which is generally 25, 30, or 60 fps.

The key insight that was employed here to overcome this problem is that in the short time slot between two FCN segmentations, the tool remains roughly rigid and its appearance changes can be captured sufficiently well by an affine transformation. This type of transformation provides a trade-off between representing small changes and being robust enough for fast fitting purposes. Based on this assumption, tracking is used to detect the small motion between the last FCN-segmented frame and the current one. By registering the last FCN-segmented frame (as opposed to the most recently segmented frame) with the current one, we avoid the time-consuming feature point extraction in every frame and potentially reduce the propagation of error across frames.

Our asynchronous pipeline is illustrated in Fig. 4. The FCN segmenter runs asynchronously to the rest of the pipeline. That is, when a frame is read from the video feed, it is sent to the FCN segmenter only if the FCN is not currently busy processing a previous frame. When the FCN finishes a segmentation, it updates the *last* segmentation mask, which is stored in synchronised memory. Furthermore, the image just segmented is converted to grayscale (as matching feature points is faster than in colour images) and stored along with some (maximum 4000) foreground feature points for later use by the optical flow tracker. The feature points used are corners provided by the GoodFeaturesToTrack extractor (OPENCV implementation of the Shi-Tomasi corner detector [25]), which in combination with optical flow forms a widely successful tracking framework used for temporal constraints that satisfies our real-time requirement. All the output segmentations are computed according to the following process. First, pyramidal Lukas-Kanade [26] optical flow is employed to find the correspondence between the foreground points in the previous FCN-segmented frame and the current received frame. Then the affine transformation between the two sets of points is estimated by solving the linear least squares problem

$$\boldsymbol{A}^*, \mathbf{t}^* := \operatorname*{argmin}_{\boldsymbol{A}, \mathbf{t}} \left(\sum_{i \, \in \, \text{inliers}} \|\mathbf{n}[i] - \boldsymbol{A}\,\mathbf{p}[i] - \mathbf{t}\|^2 \right)$$

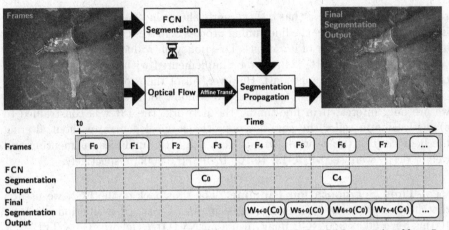

Cx: FCN Segmentation of frame Fx.
Wy←x(Cx): Warp of the segmentation Cx using the affine transformation from Fx to Fy.

Fig. 4. Real-time segmentation diagram and timeline. For the first few frames no FCN-based segmentation is available, hence the system does not provide any output. As soon as the first FCN output is retrieved, the system provides a segmentation per video frame. All the segmentation outputs **W** were obtained based on the last FCN-based output **C**.

with a RANSAC approach (`estimateRigidTransform`, OPENCV implementation to compute an optimal affine transformation between two 2D point sets) where i is the iterator over the inlier feature-point matches, $\mathbf{p}$ is the set of points in the last FCN-segmented frame, $\mathbf{n}$ is the set of points in the frame that we are currently trying to segment and $[\mathbf{A}|\mathbf{t}]$ is the affine transformation between the two sets of points that we are estimating.

Once the affine transformation is obtained, it is applied to the *last* segmentation mask produced by the FCN. This warped label is the final segmentation for the frame.

3   Experiments and Results

With the aim of demonstrating the flexibility of the presented methodology, three datasets have been used for validation. They contain training and test data for a wide variety of surgical settings, including *in vivo* abdominal and neurological surgery and different set-ups of *ex vivo* robotic surgery. Furthermore, they also contain different surgical instruments, i.e. rigid, articulated and flexible, respectively.

EndoVisSub [27]. MICCAI 2015 Endoscopic Vision Challenge - Instrument Segmentation and Tracking Sub-challenge. This dataset consists of two sub-datasets, *robotic* and *non-robotic*. The training data for the *robotic* sub-dataset is formed by four *ex vivo* 45-second videos and the test data is formed by four 15-second and two 60-second videos. All of them having a resolution of 720×576

and 25 fps. The training data for the *non-robotic* sub-dataset is formed by 160 *in vivo* abdominal images (coming from four different sequences) and the test data is formed by 4600 images (coming from nine different sequences). All of them having a resolution of 640×480. No quantitative results are reported for the non-robotic `EndoVisSub` sub-dataset as ground-truth was not available from the challenge website.

`NeuroSurgicalTools` [1]. This dataset consists of 2476 monocular images (1221 for training and 1255 for testing) coming from *in vivo* neurosurgeries. The resolution of the images varies from 612×460 to 1920×1080.

`FetalFlexTool`. *Ex vivo* fetal surgery dataset consisting of 21 images for training and a video sequence of 10 s for testing. In both the images and the video a non-rigid McKibben artificial muscle [5] is actuated close to the surface of a human placenta. In order to prove the generalisation capabilities of the method, the training images were captured in air and the video was recorded under water, to facilitate different backgrounds and lighting conditions. The ground truth of both the training images and the testing video was produced through manual segmentation. The *ex vivo* placenta used to generate this dataset was collected following a caesarean section delivery and after obtaining a written informed consent from the mother at University College London Hospitals (UCLH). The Joint UCL/UCLH Committees on Ethics of Human Research approved the study.

We implemented our method in C++, making use of the CAFFE-FUTURE branch, acceleration from the NVIDIA CUDA Deep Neural Network library v4, using the Intel(R) Math Kernel Library as BLAS choice and the CUDA module of OPENCV 3.1. The results have been generated with an Intel(R) Xeon(R) (CPU) E5-1650 v3 @ 3.50 GHz computer and a GeForce GTX TITAN X (GPU). All the results reported were obtained by fine-tuning the FCN for each dataset.

The first experiment carried out analysed the feasibility of FCN-based semantic labelling for instrument segmentation tasks without considerations for real-time requirements. The quantitative results can be seen in Table 1 and some segmentation examples are shown in Fig. 5 and the supplementary material. As can be seen in Table 1, the balanced accuracy = (sensitivity + specificity)/2 achieved for the *in vivo* `NeuroSurgicalTools` dataset is 89.6%, which is higher than the 85.8% reported by [1].

Table 1. Non-real-time quantitative results of the FCN-based segmentations. The results have been calculated based on the semantic labelling obtained for the testing images of each dataset. Three different FCN (one per dataset) have been fine-tuned to obtain these results.

Dataset	Sensitivity	Specificity	Balanced accuracy
`EndoVisSub (robotic)`	72.2%	95.2%	83.7%
`NeuroSurgicalTools`	82.0%	97.2%	89.6%
`FetalFlexTool`	84.6%	99.9%	92.3%

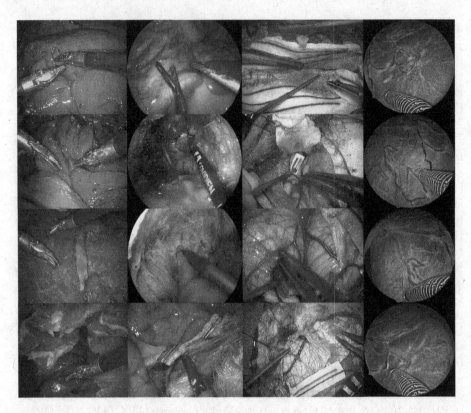

Fig. 5. FCN-based segmentation of four testing images, each one belonging to a different dataset. From left to right, `EndoVisSub (robotic)`, `EndoVisSub (non-robotic)`, `NeuroSurgicalTools` (see [1] Fig. 5 for a qualitative comparison) and `FetalFlexTool`.

Table 2. Quantitative results of the full real-time segmentation pipeline. The reported numbers are based on the frame-by-frame comparison of the binary labels provided by the presented real-time method and the ground truth video segmentations (for those datasets which have it).

Dataset	Sensitivity	Specificity	Balanced accuracy
`EndoVisSub (robotic)`	87.8%	88.7%	88.3%
`FetalFlexTool`	36.3%	99.9%	68.1%

The real-time pipeline, including the mask propagation based on optical flow, was evaluated on `EndoVisSub (robotic)` and `FetalFlexTool` (no real-time results are reported for `NeuroSurgicalTools` due to lack of frame-by-frame video ground-truth). Quantitative results can be seen in Table 2. The real-time pipeline captures the tool with a performance which is acceptable in comparison

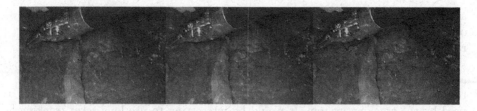

Fig. 6. Comparison between FCN-based segmentation and tracking-based propagation. From left to right, previous frame segmented with FCN (C_x), current frame segmented with FCN (C_y) and tracking-based propagation $(W_{y \leftarrow x}(C_x))$.

to the off-line counterpart, as illustrated in Fig. 6 and the supplementary material. Our method was able to produce real-time ($\approx$30 Hz) results for all the datasets.

4   Discussion and Conclusion

FCN stand out as a very promising technology for labelling endoscopic images. They can be fine-tuned with a small amount of medical images and no discriminative features have to be hand-crafted. Furthermore, these advantages are not at the expense of lowering the segmentation performance.

To the best of our knowledge this paper presents the first real-time FCN-based surgical tool labelling framework. Optical flow tracking can be successfully employed to propagate FCN segmentations in real-time. However, the quality of the results depends on how deformable the instruments being segmented are and how fast they move, as can be observed in the different results reported in Table 2. The balanced accuracy achieved by the FCN-based labelling of the EndoVisSub (robotic) dataset (83.7%) is lower than the one achieved by the real-time version (88.3%). The increase in balanced accuracy from the FCN-based segmentation to the real-time version for the EndoVisSub is at the expense of a reduction in specificity. This is due to an inflation of the warped segmentation and related to the fact that several tools are present in the foreground and move in different directions. This may benefit the accuracy score by increasing sensitivity, similar effects have been observed for anchor box trackers (votchallenge.net). For the FetalFlexTool dataset which consists of a flexible McKibben actuator the balanced accuracy was reduced from 92.3% to 68.1%.

According to the results reported for the different datasets, we can conclude that the presented methodology is flexible enough to easily adapt to different clinical scenarios. Furthermore, feasibility for real-time segmentation of different surgical instruments has been demonstrated. This including non-rigid tools, as it is the case in the FetalFlexTool dataset.

However, as it would be expected, non-rigid foreground movements (either caused by the presence of several instruments or due to genuine non-rigid tool movements) that are faster than the time elapsed between two FCN segmentations (typically 100 ms) affect the segmentation quality and will not be captured as well. This could be further addressed by separating the feature points detected on the foreground in different groups and using a set of affine transformations rather than a single one for the whole foreground.

Future work includes the possibility of detecting multiple instruments and also the inclusion of a Tracking Learning Detection framework [28]. At this stage, temporal information of previous segmentations is not fed to the FCN but is only used by the tracking system. It would be interesting to use long-term tracking information to both speed-up and improve the segmentation results.

Acknowledgements. This work was supported by Wellcome Trust [WT101957], EPSRC (NS/A000027/1, EP/H046410/1, EP/J020990/1, EP/K005278), NIHR BRC UCLH/UCL High Impact Initiative and a UCL EPSRC CDT Scholarship Award (EP/L016478/1). The authors would like to thank NVIDIA for the donated GeForce GTX TITAN X GPU, their colleagues E. Maneas, S. Moriconi, F. Chadebecq, M. Ebner and S. Nousias for the ground truth of **FetalFlexTool** and E. Maneas for preparing setup with an *ex vivo* placenta.

References

1. Bouget, D., Benenson, R., Omran, M., Riffaud, L., Schiele, B., Jannin, P.: Detecting surgical tools by modelling local appearance and global shape. IEEE Trans. Med. Imaging **34**(12), 2603–2617 (2015)
2. Daga, P., Chadebecq, F., Shakir, D., Garcia-Peraza Herrera, L.C., Tella, M., Dwyer, G., David, A.L., Deprest, J., Stoyanov, D., Vercauteren, T., Ourselin, S.: Real-time mosaicing of fetoscopic videos using SIFT. In: SPIE Medical Imaging (2015)
3. Sznitman, R., Ali, K., Richa, R., Taylor, R.H., Hager, G.D., Fua, P.: Data-driven visual tracking in retinal microsurgery. In: Ayache, N., Delingette, H., Golland, P., Mori, K. (eds.) MICCAI 2012. LNCS, vol. 7511, pp. 568–575. Springer, Heidelberg (2012). doi:10.1007/978-3-642-33418-4_70
4. Tella, M., Daga, P., Chadebecq, F., Thompson, S., Shakir, D., Dwyer, G., Wimalasundera, R., Deprest, J., Stoyanov, D., Vercauteren, T., Ourselin, S.: A combined EM and visual tracking probabilistic model for robust mosaicking of fetoscopic videos. In: IWBIR (2016)
5. Devreker, A., Rosa, B., Desjardins, A., Alles, E., Garcia-Peraza, L., Maneas, E., Stoyanov, D., David, A., Vercauteren, T., Deprest, J., Ourselin, S., Reynaerts, D., Vander Poorten, E.: Fluidic actuation for intra-operative in situ imaging. In: IROS, pp. 1415–1421. IEEE (2015)
6. Reiter, A., Allen, P.K., Zhao, T.: Marker-less articulated surgical tool detection. In: CARS (2012)
7. Allan, M., Ourselin, S., Thompson, S., Hawkes, D.J., Kelly, J., Stoyanov, D.: Toward detection and localization of instruments in minimally invasive surgery. IEEE Trans. Biomed. Eng. **60**(4), 1050–1058 (2013)
8. Allan, M., Thompson, S., Clarkson, M.J., Ourselin, S., Hawkes, D.J., Kelly, J., Stoyanov, D.: 2D-3D pose tracking of rigid instruments in minimally invasive surgery. In: Stoyanov, D., Collins, D.L., Sakuma, I., Abolmaesumi, P., Jannin, P. (eds.) IPCAI 2014. LNCS, vol. 8498, pp. 1–10. Springer, Cham (2014). doi:10.1007/978-3-319-07521-1_1

9. Pezzementi, Z., Voros, S., Hager, G.D.: Articulated object tracking by rendering consistent appearance parts. In: ICRA, pp. 3940–3947. IEEE (2009)
10. Reiter, A., Goldman, R.E., Bajo, A., Iliopoulos, K., Simaan, N., Allen, P.K.: A learning algorithm for visual pose estimation of continuum robots. In: IROS, pp. 2390–2396. IEEE, September 2011
11. Voros, S., Orvain, E., Cinquin, P., Long, J.A.: Automatic detection of instruments in laparoscopic images: a first step towards high level command of robotized endoscopic holders. In: The First IEEE/RAS-EMBS International Conference on Biomedical Robotics and Biomechatronics (BioRob 2006), pp. 1107–1112. IEEE (2006)
12. Reiter, A., Allen, P.K., Zhao, T.: Appearance learning for 3D tracking of robotic surgical tools. Int. J. Robot. Res. **33**(2), 342–356 (2014)
13. Girshick, R.: Fast R-CNN. In: ICCV, pp. 1440–1448 (2015)
14. Ren, S., He, K., Girshick, R., Sun, J.: Faster R-CNN: towards real-time object detection with region proposal networks, pp. 1–9 (2015)
15. Everingham, M., Van Gool, L., Williams, C.K.I., Winn, J., Zisserman, A.: The PASCAL VOC Challenge 2007 Results. http://www.pascal-network.org/challenges/VOC/voc2007/workshop/index.html
16. Twinanda, A.P., Shehata, S., Mutter, D., Marescaux, J., de Mathelin, M., Padoy, N.: EndoNet: a deep architecture for recognition tasks on laparoscopic videos. In: CVPR, pp. 1–10 (2016)
17. Fetoscope: https://www.karlstorz.com/doc/interactivebrochure/3317862/html5
18. Noh, H., Hong, S., Han, B.: Learning deconvolution network for semantic segmentation. In: ICCV, pp. 1520–1528 (2015)
19. Long, J., Shelhamer, E., Darrell, T.: Fully convolutional networks for semantic segmentation. In: CVPR, pp. 3431–3440. IEEE (2015)
20. Krizhevsky, A., Sutskever, I., Hinton, G.E.: ImageNet classification with deep convolutional neural networks. In: NIPS, pp. 1097–1105 (2012)
21. Guerra, E., de Lara, J., Malizia, A., Díaz, P.: Supporting user-oriented analysis for multi-view domain-specific visual languages. Inf. Softw. Technol. **51**(4), 769–784 (2009)
22. Caffe Model Zoo. http://github.com/BVLC/caffe/wiki/Model-Zoo
23. Mottaghi, R., Chen, X., Liu, X., Cho, N.G., Lee, S.W., Fidler, S., Urtasun, R., Yuille, A.: The role of context for object detection and semantic segmentation in the wild. In: CVPR (2014)
24. Smith, L.N.: No more pesky learning rate guessing games. Arxiv, June 2015
25. Shi, J., Tomasi, C.: Good features to track. In: IEEE Computer Society Conference on CVPR, pp. 593–600 (1994)
26. Bouguet, J.Y.: Pyramidal implementation of the lucas kanade feature tracker: description of the algorithm. Technical report, Intel Corporation Microprocessor Research Labs (2000)
27. MICCAI. http://endovissub-instrument.grand-challenge.org
28. Kalal, Z., Mikolajczyk, K., Matas, J.: Tracking-learning-detection. IEEE Trans. Pattern Anal. Mach. Intell. **34**(7), 1409–1422 (2012)

Weakly-Supervised Lesion Detection in Video Capsule Endoscopy Based on a Bag-of-Colour Features Model

Michael Vasilakakis[1(✉)], Dimitrios K. Iakovidis[1], Evaggelos Spyrou[2],
and Anastasios Koulaouzidis[3]

[1] Department of Computer Science and Biomedical Informatics, University of Thessaly,
Lamia, Greece
vasilaka.inf@gmail.com, dimitris.iakovidis@ieee.org
[2] National Center for Scientific Research - Demokritos, Institute of Informatics
and Telecommunications, Athens, Greece
espyrou@iit.demokritos.gr
[3] Endoscopy Unit, The Royal Infirmary of Edinburgh, Edinburgh, UK
akoulaouzidis@hotmail.com

Abstract. Robotic video capsule endoscopy (VCE) is a rapidly evolving medical imaging technology enabling more thorough examination and treatment of the gastrointestinal tract than conventional endoscopy technologies. Despite of the technological advances in this field, the reviewing of the large VCE image sequences remains manual and challenges experts' diagnostic capabilities. Video reviewing systems for automated lesion detection are still under investigation. Most of these systems are based on supervised machine learning algorithms, which require a training set of images, manually annotated by the experts to indicate which pixels correspond to lesions. In this paper, we investigate a weakly-supervised approach for lesion detection, which requires image-level instead of pixel-level annotations for training. Such an approach offers a considerable advantage with respect to the efficiency of the annotation process. It is based on state-of-the-art colour features, which, in this study, are extended according to the bag-of-visual-words model. The area under receiver operating characteristic achieved, reaches 81%.

Keywords: Video capsule endoscopy · Lesion detection · Colour features · Bag-of-Words · Weakly-supervised learning

1 Introduction

Video capsule endoscopy (VCE) enables the examination of the whole gastrointestinal (GI) tract in a non-invasive way. It is performed with a swallowable capsule endoscope (CE), which captures colour images during its approx. 12 h battery lifetime. Today's commercial CEs are passive, in the sense that they are moving by exploiting both the gravity and the peristaltic motion of the GI tract. However, several research prototypes have been proposed for active, robotic capsule endoscopy, which will enable thorougher examinations, easier lesion localization, and drug infusion [1].

© Springer International Publishing AG 2017
T. Peters et al. (Eds.): CARE 2016, LNCS 10170, pp. 96–103, 2017.
DOI: 10.1007/978-3-319-54057-3_9

A major issue that is still unresolved, both in passive and active VCE is that it requires a lot of human effort for manually reviewing of the produced videos. Typically, each individual review lasts 45–90 min, during which, the reviewer's concentration should remain undivided for a careful inspection of the output video [2]. Such a tiring procedure is prone to human errors; a fact with serious consequences in the diagnostic yield, which is alarmingly low [3].

In order to cope with this problem, automated lesion detection methods based on computer vision algorithms have been proposed [4]. Most of these methods exploit supervised machine learning methodologies, capable of learning what is defined as normal and what is defined as an abnormal finding within the VCE video. The generation of datasets for training the learning machines requires that experts indicate which pixels correspond to normal or abnormal tissues within the VCE images. Considering that the videos produced by a VCE examination are composed of thousands of frames (usually of the order of 10^4), such a pixel-wise annotation task can prove very time-consuming and discouraging for annotation of large datasets by the experts.

A promising solution that could alleviate this problem is weakly-supervised learning, which involves training of a learning machine using weakly annotated data [5, 6]. In this paper weakly supervised learning is considered using images annotated at image-level instead of pixel-level. This way, a binary semantic label is assigned per video frame indicating whether its content is normal or abnormal. A drawback of such an approach is that the abnormal images can be tracked, but the localization of the lesion(s) within each abnormal frame remains a challenge. However, it is much more significant for the system to robustly detect which frames contain possible lesions than to localize the lesion within these frames, since this can be much easier done by the video reviewers.

The Bag-of-Words or Bag-of-Visual Words (BoW/BoVW) can be considered as a weakly supervised model built upon the notion of visual vocabularies. A visual vocabulary may be seen as a set of "exemplar" image patches (visual words), in terms of which any given image may be described. Typically, this vocabulary is built using a large corpus of representative images of the domain of interest and should be closely related to the problem at hand. The vocabulary may be seen as a means of quantization of the feature space i.e., the one of the local descriptors. Any unseen descriptor may then be easily quantized to its nearest visual word. The description of the whole image is formed by a histogram, counting the appearances of each visual word within it. Apart from the obvious advantage of BoW, i.e., that can be used as a weakly supervised approach as it has already been discussed, it also provides a fixed-size representation, a useful property for tasks such as classification using traditional classifiers e.g., feed-forward neural networks, support vector machines etc. Finally, the visual description provided by BoW may also be used on tasks such as inverted file indexing [7], visual retrieval etc.

An early application of BoW in capsule endoscopy has been investigated using speeded-up robust features (SURF) for polyp detection [8]. In [9] the performance of BoW was investigated using scale-invariant feature transform features (SIFT) and local binary patterns (LBP) for ulcer detection. A more complex feature extraction scheme for the construction required in BoW was proposed in [10]. This scheme was applied for polyp detection and includes extraction of SIFT, LBP, uniform LBP and histogram of oriented gradients (HoG) features from neighbourhoods of salient points detected using the SIFT key-point detector. In the context of bleeding detection, colour histograms extracted from various colour spaces were considered [11]. Colour along with textural information has also been exploited in [12] for detection of gastric and oesophageal cancer, gastritis, and oesophagitis. In that study superpixel segmentation was exploited for estimation of image descriptors from homogeneous regions. As in [12] the descriptors considered include colour histograms from various colour spaces as well as LBP-based textural signatures. Most of the aforementioned approaches are based on support vector machine (SVM) classifiers.

The BoW model was also exploited in the context of unsupervised segmentation of capsule endoscopy videos, based on probabilistic latent semantic analysis (pLSA) [13]. In the context of the analysis of higher resolution endoscopic images, BoW models have been proposed for browsing endoscopic imagery by semantic information [14], colonoscopy image classification [15], and classification of images obtained using chromoendoscopy and narrow-band imaging techniques.

Acknowledging the significance of incorporating an image-level instead of pixel-level annotation process in the development of training datasets for lesion detection systems in VCE, in this paper we investigate a novel BoW-based weakly-supervised learning approach using the state-of-the-art features that have been proposed in [15]. These features represent colour information both at pixel and region level in CIE-*Lab* colour space, and despite their simplicity they have been proved very effective in the detection of a diverse set of abnormalities [5, 17].

The rest of this paper is organized as follows: In Sect. 2 we describe the methodology we followed for the proposed weakly supervised classification scheme. We provide a brief description of both the generic BoW methodology and the approach we followed. Then, in Sect. 3 we demonstrate and discuss our experimental results. Finally, conclusions are drawn in Sect. 4, where we also discuss plans for future continuation of this work.

2   Methodology

BoW is a widely used method to model generic categories in detection, classification and recognition problems [18]. This method has been originally inspired by text document analysis techniques, and consists of calculating word frequencies. The first step of BoW is to describe an image as a set of "words", which capture its visual content. To this goal, given an adequately large dataset, a set of features is extracted from every image and typically quantized using a clustering approach, e.g., the k-means algorithm [19]. Upon clustering, the centroids (or in some approaches the *medoids*, which opposed to centroids are actual members of the dataset) that have been determined, are used as a "visual vocabulary" and are often referred to as "visual words."

Each feature is then translated (coded) into one of these visual words, i.e., to the nearest one in the feature space (typically based on the Euclidean distance). The next step involves a histogram construction, which describes the appearance frequency of every visual word within an image. Thus, this histogram is used to characterize the visual content of the image. Among the advantages of BoW, we should emphasize that it succeeds to reduce the problem of classifying a large number of high dimensional vectors from local point descriptors to a fixed-size, one dimensional vector without significant loss of visual information. Finally, any typical classification approach may be used for the classification of these histogram vectors. In this work we choose to use an SVM [20], trained with examples of histograms extracted from both normal and abnormal categories.

We use the well-known SURF (speeded up robust features) algorithm [21], in order to detect interest points and extract descriptions from patches around them. SURF is a powerful and fast descriptor scheme and has been successfully applied to a plethora of computer vision problems. It has been shown to achieve comparable repeatability and performance to other, more sophisticated schemes, at a lower computational cost. It combines a Hessian-Laplace region detector and a gradient orientation-based feature descriptor and is invariant to several image transformations and robust to illumination variations. For interest point selection, we also make use of a "naïve" approach known as "dense sampling". Following this approach, we select all pixels sampled using a regular grid (i.e., one with equal horizontal and vertical inter-pixel distances), which are then used as interest points. Although these points cannot be matched accurately, when compared e.g., to the SURF interest points, they carry valuable information regarding image content interpretation [22].

For the extraction of visual descriptions of patches around the interest points, we also evaluate the colour-based features of [16]. Images are first transformed to the CIE-*Lab* colour space and then, the following colour information is extracted from a square region centered at each point: (i) The *Lab* values of each interest point; (ii) The minimal and maximal values of each component. This results to a vector consisting of 9 values.

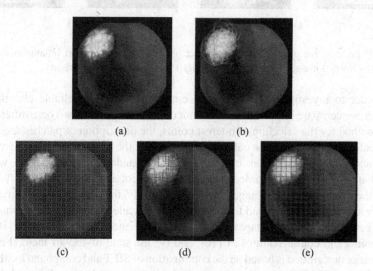

Fig. 1. Image examples of different uses of the algorithms: (a) A raw WCE image depicting lymphangiectasia; (b) SURF; (c) Dense SURF; (d) *Lab*; and (e) Dense *Lab*.

In Fig. 1(b) and (d) we illustrate the set of the SURF interest points extracted from a given VCE image, combined with SURF regions and fixed windows, respectively, whilst in Fig. 1(c) and (e) we illustrate the set of the dense interest points, also combined with SURF regions and fixed windows. One may easily observe that SURF points do not cover the visual properties of the whole image. Yet, the latter is achieved by the dense features.

3   Results

For the evaluation of the proposed weakly-supervised BoW approach, we performed experiments using a subset of dataset 2 from the publicly available KID database [23, 24]. This dataset displays a variety of different kinds of abnormalities. More precisely, the selected subset consists of 227 images of most common inflammatory lesions, e.g., as in Fig. 2(a) including ulcers, aphthae, mucosal breaks with surrounding erythema, cobblestone mucosa, stenoses and/or fibrotic strictures, and significant mucosal/villous oedema. It also includes a set of 1327 normal images derived from the small bowel (728 images), e.g., as in Fig. 2(b) (right), and the stomach (599 images), e.g., as in Fig. 2(b) (left).

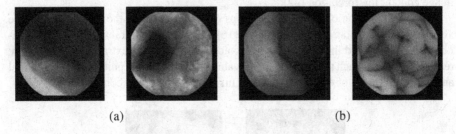

(a)   (b)

Fig. 2. Representative images from the dataset used in experiments: (a) Inflammatory lesion images, (b) Normal images from the stomach (left) and the small bowel (right)

In order to investigate whether BoW could be used as a reliable classification approach, we compare its performance in four different experiments. These differentiate on the method for the selection of interest points, the description of patches around the aforementioned points; and the colour space used. For the latter case we used greyscale images and also transformations of CIE-*Lab* (using standard illuminant D65), where L and b channels had been discarded, keeping only the colour information of a. We shall refer to the latter as the "*Lab* images". More specifically, the performed experiments are as follows: (i) SURF points and features on the greyscale image; (ii) dense points and SURF features on the *Lab* images; (iii) SURF points and colour features of [16]; (iv) dense points and colour features of [16]; and (v) the state-of-the-art method of [10], where image description is based on the combination of SIFT and compound local binary pattern features (CLBP). In each case, we extract interest points, then their descriptions, we create the visual vocabulary, which we use for image BoW description and finally train SVM classifiers. In every experiment we use 6-fold cross validation method and estimate the values of area under the receiver operating characteristic (AUC).

The visual vocabulary size ranged from 300 to 1200 words. For the experiments with dense SURF, we used multi-scale feature extraction with scale step 1.6, starting from scale 1.6, up to scale 6.4. We also experimented with various sizes of square regions, for the extraction of the colour features. We used 18 × 18 and 36 × 36 square areas. For dense feature extraction we used grid steps of 4, 10, 18 and 36 pixels, both horizontally and vertically. For the method of [10] we used CLBP of patch size 4 × 4 and 8 × 8. For the classification we used an SVM with RBF kernel.

Most notable results are summarized in Table 1. In this Table we may observe that best performance was achieved for the case of dense *Lab* features using a window size of 18 × 18 pixels and a visual vocabulary of 700 words. The best performance of standard SURF features (i.e., applied on grayscale images) was achieved using dense extraction and a vocabulary size of 800 words. However, this advantageous performance comes at cost of efficiency, since the number of samples obtained by dense SURF is higher (due to the regular sampling process). In addition, our approach had better results in comparison with of the state-of-the-art method of [10]. In any case the application of SURF on the *a* channel of CIE-*Lab* leads to an increase of AUC.

Table 1. Experimental Results; in dense (x), x denotes the step, in SURF (y), y denotes the colour space (g: greyscale, *a*: *a* channel of *Lab*). Note that in case of SURF feature description, image patches are selected by the algorithm, thus marked herein as "N/A"

Feature extraction	Feature description	Window size	Vocabulary size	AUC
dense (18)	*Lab* [15]	18 × 18	500	0.80
dense (4)	SURF (g)	N/A	800	0.70
dense (36)	*Lab* [15]	36 × 36	700	0.79
dense (18)	SURF (g)	18 × 18	800	0.69
dense (10)	*Lab* [15]	18 × 18	700	**0.81**
SURF (*a*)	*Lab* [15]	N/A	700	0.77
SURF (g)	SURF (g)	N/A	500	0.59
SIFT (g)	SIFT + CLBP [10]	4 × 4	500	0.73
SIFT (g)	SIFT + CLBP [10]	8 × 8	500	0.73
SIFT (g)	SIFT + CLBP [10]	8 × 8	700	0.74

4   Conclusions

In this paper we presented a weakly supervised classification scheme for automated lesion detection in VCE videos. We followed the BoW paradigm and created a visual dictionary encoding all extracted image features into visual words. A novel contribution of this paper is that we extended our state-of-the-art colour features [16, 17], according to the bag-of-visual-words model and created BoW image descriptions, which were used to train SVM classifiers. We evaluated four different feature extraction schemes, including a state-of-the-art approach, and investigated among others the use of colour and different sampling schemes. Our results indicate that standard SURF features are not capable of providing a reliable descriptor in the given problem. However, when applied to the *Lab* colour space, their performance is boosted. The latter are able to provide valuable results within the proposed weakly-supervised scheme, which could be used as an alternative to the demanding in terms of manual annotation effort, fully-supervised, schemes.

Open research topics in the area of BoW with application to weakly-supervised lesion detection include the construction of visual vocabularies (flat vs. hierarchical approaches, predefined vs. dynamically selected sizes), the selection of interest points (dense vs. salient vs. hybrid), the selection of patches surrounding interest points (shape, size, orientation) and of course their description (colour vs. greyscale vs. binary descriptors). We plan to perform a thorough systematic investigation to assess the effect of each part of BoW schemes to the overall results, within the context of lesion detection in VCE videos.

Acknowledgements. This research was supported by the special account of research grants of the Technological Educational Institute of Central Greece, Lamia, Greece.

References

1. Koulaouzidis, A., Iakovidis, D.K., Karargyris, A., Rondonotti, E.: Wireless endoscopy in 2020: Will it still be a capsule? World J. Gastroenterol. (WJG) **21**, 5119 (2015)
2. Koulaouzidis, A., Iakovidis, D.K., Karargyris, A., Plevris, J.N.: Optimizing lesion detection in small-bowel capsule endoscopy: from present problems to future solutions. Expert Rev. Gastroenterol. Hepatol. **9**, 217–235 (2015)
3. Zheng, Y., Hawkins, L., Wolff, J., Goloubeva, O., Goldberg, E.: Detection of lesions during capsule endoscopy: physician performance is disappointing. Am. J. Gastroenterol. **107**, 554–560 (2012)
4. Iakovidis, D.K., Koulaouzidis, A.: Software for enhanced video capsule endoscopy: challenges for essential progress. Nature Rev. Gastroenterol. Hepatol. **12**, 172–186 (2015)
5. Hoai, M., Torresani, L., la Torre, F.D., Rother, C.: Learning discriminative localization from weakly labeled data. Pattern Recogn. **47**, 1523–1534 (2014)
6. Blaschko, M., Vedaldi, A., Zisserman, A.: Simultaneous object detection and ranking with weak supervision. In: Advances in Neural Information Processing systems, pp. 235–243 (2010)
7. Philbin, J., Chum, O., Isard, M., Sivic, J., Zisserman, A.: Object retrieval with large vocabularies and fast spatial matching. In: proceedings of IEEE Conference on Computer Vision and Pattern Recognition, pp. 1–8. IEEE (2007)
8. Hwang, S.: Bag-of-visual-words approach based on SURF features to polyp detection in wireless capsule endoscopy videos. In: Proceedings of the 7th International Conference on Advances in Visual Computing (ISVC 2011), vol. 2, pp. 320–327 (2011)
9. Yu, L., Yuen, P.C., Lai, J.: Ulcer detection in wireless capsule endoscopy images. In: ICPR 2012, pp. 45–48. IEEE (2012)
10. Yuan, Y., Li, B., Meng, M.Q.-H.: Improved bag of feature for automatic polyp detection in wireless capsule endoscopy images. IEEE Trans. Autom. Sci. Eng. **13**, 529–535 (2016)
11. Yuan, Y., Li, B., Meng, M.Q.-H.: Bleeding frame and region detection in the wireless capsule endoscopy video. IEEE J. Biomed. Health Inf. **20**, 624–630 (2016)
12. Wang, S., et al.: Computer-aided endoscopic diagnosis without human specific labeling. IEEE Trans. Bio Med. Eng. **53**(11), 2347–2358 (2016)

13. Shen, Y., Guturu, P., Buckles, B.P.: Wireless capsule endoscopy video segmentation using an unsupervised learning approach based on probabilistic latent semantic analysis with scale invariant features. IEEE Trans. Inf Technol. Biomed. **16**, 98–105 (2012)

14. Kwitt, R., Vasconcelos, N., Rasiwasia, N., Uhl, A., Davis, B., Häfner, M., Wrba, F.: Endoscopic image analysis in semantic space. Med. Image Anal. **16**, 1415–1422 (2012)

15. Manivannan, S., Trucco, E.: Learning discriminative local features from image-level labelled data for colonoscopy image classification. In: 2015 IEEE 12th International Symposium on Biomedical Imaging (ISBI), pp. 420–423. IEEE (2015)

16. Iakovidis, D.K., Koulaouzidis, A.: Automatic lesion detection in capsule endoscopy based on color saliency: closer to an essential adjunct for reviewing software. Gastrointest. Endosc. **80**, 877–883 (2014)

17. Iakovidis, D.K., Koulaouzidis, A.: Automatic lesion detection in wireless capsule endoscopy - a simple solution for a complex problem. In: 2014 IEEE International Conference on Image Processing (ICIP), pp. 2236–2240. IEEE (2014)

18. Sivic, J., Zisserman, A.: Efficient visual search of videos cast as text retrieval. IEEE Trans. Pattern Anal. Mach. Intell. **31**(4), 591–606 (2009)

19. Drake, J., Hamerly, G.: Accelerated k-means with adaptive distance bounds. In: 5th NIPS Workshop on Optimization for Machine Learning (2012)

20. Burges, C.J.: A tutorial on support vector machines for pattern recognition. Data Min. Knowl. Disc. **2**(2), 121–167 (1998)

21. Bay, H., Ess, A., Tuytelaars, T., Van Gool, L.: Speeded-up robust features (SURF). Comput. Vis. Image Underst. **110**(3), 346–359 (2008)

22. Tuytelaars, T.: Dense interest points. In: 2010 IEEE Conference on Proceedings of IEEE Conference on Computer Vision and Pattern Recognition (CVPR), pp. 2281–2288. IEEE (2010)

23. Iakovidis, D.K., Koulaouzidis, A.: Software for enhanced video capsule endoscopy: challenges for essential progress. Nature Rev. Gastroenterol. Hepatol. **12**(3), 172–186 (2015)

24. Koulaouzidis, A., Iakovidis, D.K.: KID: Koulaouzidis-Iakovidis database for capsule endoscopy (2015). http://is-innovation.eu/kid

Convolutional Neural Network Architectures for the Automated Diagnosis of Celiac Disease

G. Wimmer[1]([✉]), S. Hegenbart[1], A. Vecsei[2], and A. Uhl[1]

[1] Department of Computer Sciences, University of Salzburg, Salzburg, Austria
gwimmer@cosy.sbg.ac.at
[2] Department Pediatrics, St. Anna Children's Hospital, Vienna, Austria

Abstract. In this work, convolutional neural networks (CNNs) are applied for the computer assisted diagnosis of celiac disease based on endoscopic images of the duodenum. To evaluate which network configurations are best suited for the classification of celiac disease, several different CNN networks were trained using different numbers of layers and filters and different filter dimensions. The results of the CNNs are compared with the results of popular general purpose image representations such as Improved Fisher Vectors and LBP-based methods as well as a feature representations especially designed for the classification of celiac disease. We will show that the deeper CNN architectures outperform these comparison approaches and that combining CNNs with linear support vector machines furtherly improves the classification rates for about 3–7% leading to distinctly better results (up to 97%) than those of the comparison methods.

Keywords: CNN · Celiac disease · Endoscopy · Deep learning

1 Introduction

Convolutional neural networks (CNN) are gaining more and more interest in computer vision. The increase in computational power based on GPUs has led to more sophisticated and deeper architectures which have proven in various challenges to be the state-of-the art in image classification. Generally thousands or millions of images are used and required as data corpus to achieve well generalizing deep architectures. In endoscopic image classification however the available amount of data usable as training corpus is often much more limited to a few hundreds or thousands of images or even less. Another difference to datasets such as used in ILSVRC or Places is however that image classification problems in medical scenarios are often reduced to a few categories instead of thousands in the former. Consequently, deep architectures designed for recognizing images from thousands of categories could be too complex for the classification of celiac disease.

CNNs are already widely used for the computer aided diagnosis in medical scenarios [10], however not so in the computer aided diagnosis using endoscopic

© Springer International Publishing AG 2017
T. Peters et al. (Eds.): CARE 2016, LNCS 10170, pp. 104–113, 2017.
DOI: 10.1007/978-3-319-54057-3_10

imagery. We found only three publications in this area, 2 about the classification of digestive organs using wireless capsule endoscopy images [19,21] and one about lesion detection [20] in endoscopic images. Since the classification of celiac disease can be considered as a texture classification problem and CNNs are state-of-the-art in texture recognition, CNNs are promising image representations for the automated classification of celiac disease.

In this experimental study we apply CNNs for the classification of celiac disease using a experimental setup especially adapted for endoscopic imagery and we try to answer the following open questions:

1. Are deep-architectures suited to classify celiac disease or are simpler and more shallow architectures more suited in such a scenario because of the low amount of training data and categories
2. What are the best network configurations like e.g. the number or filters and their dimensions
3. How well do CNNs perform compared to other state-of-the-art approaches
4. Are linear support vector machines (SVMs) able to furtherly improve the results when applied on the activations of the nets.

2   Celiac Disease

Celiac disease is a complex autoimmune disorder in genetically predisposed individuals of all age groups after introduction of gluten containing food. The gastrointestinal manifestations invariably comprise an inflammatory reaction within the mucosa of the small intestine caused by a dysregulated immune response triggered by ingested gluten protein. During the course of the disease, hyperplasia of the enteric crypts occurs and the mucosa eventually looses its absorptive villi thus leading to a diminished ability to absorb nutrients. [5] state that more than 2 million people in the United States, this is about one in 133, have the disease. People with untreated celiac disease are at risk for developing various complications like osteoporosis, infertility and other autoimmune diseases including type 1 diabetes, autoimmune thyroid disease and autoimmune liver disease. So an early diagnosis is of highest importance.

Endoscopy with biopsy is currently considered the gold standard for the diagnosis of celiac disease. Computer-assisted systems for the diagnosis of CD have potential to improve the whole diagnostic work-up, by saving costs, time and manpower and at the same time increase the safety of the procedure. A motivation for such a system is furthermore given as the inter-observer variability is reported to be high [1,12]. A survey on computer aided decision support for the diagnosis of celiac disease can be found in [9].

Besides standard upper endoscopy, several new endoscopic approaches for diagnosing CD have been evaluated and found their way into clinical practice [2]. The most notable techniques include the modified immersion technique (MIT [7]) under traditional white-light illumination (denoted as WL_{MIT}), as well as MIT

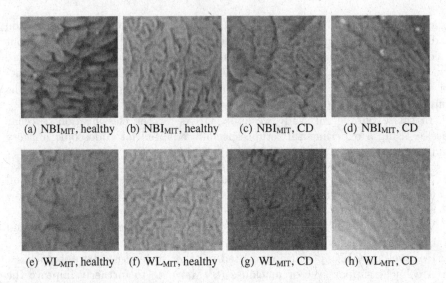

(a) NBI$_{MIT}$, healthy   (b) NBI$_{MIT}$, healthy   (c) NBI$_{MIT}$, CD   (d) NBI$_{MIT}$, CD

(e) WL$_{MIT}$, healthy   (f) WL$_{MIT}$, healthy   (g) WL$_{MIT}$, CD   (h) WL$_{MIT}$, CD

Fig. 1. Example images for the two classes healthy and celiac disease (CD) using NBI$_{MIT}$ as well as WL$_{MIT}$ endoscopy

under narrow band imaging [3,17] (denoted as NBI$_{MIT}$). These specialized endoscopic techniques were specifically designed for improving the visual confirmation of CD during endoscopy.

In this work we differentiate between healthy mucosa and mucosa affected by celiac disease using images gathered by NBI$_{MIT}$ as well as WL$_{MIT}$ endoscopy. Examples of the two classes for both endoscopy types are shown in Fig. 1. In [6] it was shown that using NBI$_{MIT}$ or WL$_{MIT}$ as imaging modality has a significant impact on the underlying feature distribution of general purpose image representations. However, it was also shown that systems trained on images from both modalities generalize well without requiring additional domain adaption techniques and that combining both modalities improves the accuracies in case of an insufficient amount of data for training (as is probably the case for CNNs).

3   CNN Architectures

All our networks share the same basic principal architecture. They consist of a variable number of convolutional blocks (CONV) using rectified linear units (RELU) for non-linearity, local response normalization (LRN) [11] and max-pooling (POOL), two fully connected blocks (FC) using RELU and dropout and a last fully connected block acting as soft-max classifier: [CONV, RELU, LRN, POOL]^n → [FC, RELU, DROPOUT]^2 → [FC, SOFTMAXLOSS]. We only vary the number of convolutional blocks, the filter dimensions and the number of filters. To provide a systematic analysis, we trained networks with $n = 1, 2, 3$ and 4 convolutional blocks using different filter dimensions and different numbers of filters in each layer. We follow the general approach of employing large filter dimensions in lower layers and subsequently smaller filters in higher layers.

A high number of filters per layer allows the training process to adapt to highly abstract features. However, it is unclear in the context of celiac disease and endoscopic imagery in general if such abstract features are visible or even useful for prediction. Consequently, we analyze the impact of the number of filters per layer by training multiple nets of the same architecture with varying numbers of filters. We generally rely on the concept of increasing the number of filters from the lower to the higher layers by a factor of two per layer.

All our models are initialized and trained using the same set of techniques. The coefficients of the nets are randomly initialized based on He et al. [8] and the bias terms are initialized as 0. All architectures rely on using max-pooling with a windows size of three and stride two. Stochastic gradient descent (SGD) with weight decay ($\lambda = 0.0005$) and momentum ($\mu = 0.9$) is used for the training of the models. Regularization is achieved using drop-out ($p = 0.5$) during training. Training is performed on batches of 128 images each, which are for each iteration randomly chosen from the training data and subsequently augmented (see Sect. 4.1). The learning rate is initialized at 0.01 and four times divided by three whenever the training-loss stopped improving with the current learning rate. For this, each 250th iteration we compute the average loss of the previous 250 iterations. If the currently computed average loss is greater than 0.99 times the previously computed average loss and if the current learning rate is in use for at least 1000 iterations, then the learning rate is divided by three. Due to the differing number of parameters among the architectures, optimization is continued until the training-loss shows no improvement over 2500 iterations but at least until the learning rate has been reduced the fourth time. The model of the iteration achieving the lowest training-loss is then used for validation.

Our learning rate configurations and break off condition are especially adapted on our celiac disease image data to achieve high results without needing too much time for training (the nets were trained for ≈10000 iterations in average). Since we train 36 different nets (4 (different numbers of convolutional blocks) × 3 (different filter sizes) × 3 (different filter numbers)) on 10 different training splits (see Sect. 4.1), we had to choose such configurations that enable a limited time of training per network.

3.1 Very-Shallow Networks

We start off with a very uncommon variation of CNNs using only one single convolutional block. By analyzing different architectures growing from very shallow to deep we hope to gain some insight on the problem. Although this sort of architecture is quite uncommon and might not fit into the general CNN schemes, the lower abstraction of features in endoscopic images and the small number of categories (two) make it necessary to start with such shallow architectures. The Very-Shallow networks (see Table 1) are trained with $N = 10, 48$ and 96 filters to analyze the impact of the number of filters on the results.

Table 1. Architecture of the Very-Shallow networks. The first row in a convolutional block (CONV) specifies the receptive field size of the convolutional filters and their number (N). The second row indicates the stride (st.) and padding (pad). Furtherly we indicate the dimensionality of the fully connected (FC) blocks.

Filter size	CONV$_1$	FC$_1$	FC$_2$	FC$_3$
Large	$11 \times 11 \times N$ st. 3, pad 0	512 drop-out	512 drop-out	2 soft-max
Medium	$7 \times 7 \times N$ st. 3, pad 0	512 drop-out	512 drop-out	2 soft-max
Small	$5 \times 5 \times N$ st. 2, pad 0	512 drop-out	512 drop-out	2 soft-max

3.2 Shallow Networks

The next generation of architectures is based on the Very-Shallow networks but the number of convolutional blocks is increased to two. Like in the previous and also in the following deeper network architectures, the network is trained with different numbers of filters ($N = 10, 48$ and 96 filters in the first convolutional layer). The network architecture of the Shallow nets is shown in Table 2.

Table 2. Architecture of the Shallow networks.

Filter size	CONV$_1$	CONV$_2$	FC$_1$	FC$_2$	FC$_3$
Large	$11 \times 11 \times N$ st. 3, pad 0	$7 \times 7 \times 2N$ st. 3, pad 0	512 drop-out	512 drop-out	2 soft-max
Medium	$7 \times 7 \times N$ st. 4, pad 0	$5 \times 5 \times 2N$ st. 2, pad 0	512 drop-out	512 drop-out	2 soft-max
Small	$5 \times 5 \times N$ st. 3, pad 0	$3 \times 3 \times 2N$ st. 2, pad 0	512 drop-out	512 drop-out	2 soft-max

3.3 Deep Networks

The third generation of nets use 3 convolutional blocks and can therefore be considered as our first deep architecture. The network architecture of the Deep nets is shown in Table 3.

Table 3. Architecture of the Deep networks, where $m_b^a = \max(a, b)$ and denotes the number of convolutional filters.

Filter size	CONV$_1$	CONV$_2$	CONV$_3$	FC$_1$	FC$_2$	FC$_3$
Large	$11 \times 11 \times N$ st. 2, pad 0	$7 \times 7 \times m_{2N}^{128}$ st. 1, pad 0	$5 \times 5 \times m_{4N}^{256}$ st. 1 pad 0	512 drop-out	512 drop-out	2 soft-max
Medium	$7 \times 7 \times N$ st. 2, pad 0	$5 \times 5 \times m_{2N}^{128}$ st. 1, pad 0	$3 \times 3 \times m_{4N}^{256}$ st. 1, pad 0	512 drop-out	512 drop-out	2 soft-max
Small	$5 \times 5 \times N$ st. 2, pad 0	$3 \times 3 \times m_{2N}^{128}$ st. 1, pad 0	$3 \times 3 \times m_{4N}^{256}$ st. 1, pad 0	512 drop-out	512 drop-out	2 soft-max

3.4   Very-Deep Networks

In our last generation of nets we use 4 convolutional blocks (see Table 4). Although the term Very-Deep is not quite true considering the number of layers of other very-deep architectures, we use the term to easily distinguish between our four basic architectures.

Table 4. Architecture of the Very-Deep networks, where $m_b^a = \max(a, b)$.

Filter size	CONV$_1$	CONV$_2$	CONV$_3$	CONV$_4$	FC$_1$	FC$_2$	FC$_3$
Large	$11 \times 11 \times N$ st. 1, pad 2	$7 \times 7 \times m_{2N}^{192}$ st. 1, pad 0	$5 \times 5 \times m_{4N}^{256}$ st. 1, pad 0	$3 \times 3 \times m_{8N}^{256}$ st. 1, pad 0	1024 drop-out	1024 drop-out	2 soft-max
Medium	$7 \times 7 \times N$ st. 2, pad 0	$5 \times 5 \times m_{2N}^{192}$ st. 1, pad 0	$3 \times 3 \times m_{4N}^{256}$ st. 1, pad 0	$3 \times 3 \times m_{8N}^{256}$ st. 1, pad 0	1024 drop-out	1024 drop-out	2 soft-max
Small	$5 \times 5 \times N$ st. 2, pad 0	$3 \times 3 \times m_{2N}^{192}$ st. 1, pad 0	$3 \times 3 \times m_{4N}^{256}$ st. 1, pad 0	$3 \times 3 \times m_{8N}^{256}$ st. 1, pad 0	1024 drop-out	1024 drop-out	2 soft-max

4   Experimental Setup and Results

4.1   Experimental Setup

Our celiac disease image database consists of 1661 RGB image patches of size 128×128 pixels that are gathered by means of flexible endoscopes using NBI$_{\text{MIT}}$ as well as WL$_{\text{MIT}}$. The database consists of 1045 images gathered by WL$_{\text{MIT}}$ endoscopy (587 healthy images and 458 affected by celiac disease) and 616 images gathered by NBI$_{\text{MIT}}$ endoscopy (399 healthy images and 217 affected by celiac disease). So in total 986 image patches show healthy mucosa and the remaining 675 image patches show mucosa affected by celiac disease. The images were captured from 353 patients.

Due to the relatively small amount of data, we perform cross-validation to achieve a stable estimation of the generalization error. We generated 10 (fixed) splits for training and validation (80% training and 20% validation) and took care that images of a single patient are never in training and evaluation sets. All nets are trained using the training portion of our data corpus. The final validation was performed on the left-out part.

The image data is normalized by subtracting the mean image of the training portion. We then linearly scale each image within $[-1, 1]$. Due to the small amount of available data we use data augmentation to increase the number of images for training. Augmentation is applied to the batches of images extracted for training. The augmentation is based on cropping one sub-image (112×112 pixels) from each training image with randomly chosen position. Subsequently, the sub-image is randomly rotated ($0°$, $90°$, $180°$ or $270°$) and randomly either horizontally reflected or not. Validation is performed using a majority voting of five crops from the validation image using the upper left, upper right, lower left, lower right and center part.

In our experiments, we compute the overall classification rate (OCR) for each split and report the mean OCR over all 10 splits with the respective standard deviation.

The CNNs are implemented using the *MatConvNet* framework [18]. Additionally to the CNN soft-max-classifier we employ linear SVMs as provided by the *LIBLINEAR* library [4]. For this, the training and test samples are fed through the CNNs and the output of the second fully connected layer is extracted as feature for further SVM classification. The size of the extracted feature vector per image is 1024×1 in case of the very-deep architectures and 512×1 for the other architectures. Augmentation is also applied for the extraction of features from the nets for further for SVM classification. The augmentation is basically the same as for the training of the nets with only one difference. The patches of the training images are extracted from the fixed center position instead from random positions (8 patches per image with 4 different rotations, either horizontally flipped or not). The SVM cost factor (C) is found using cross validation on the training data.

Additionally, we combine CNNs, principle component analysis (PCA) and SVMs by applying PCA to the CNN features resulting in 100 principal components which are furtherly classified using SVMs.

We compare the CNNs against three popular general purpose image representations and one feature representations especially developed for the classification of celiac disease. As general purpose image representations we use multi-resolution local binary patterns (LBP [13]) and multi-resolution local ternary patterns (LTP [15]), both with 3 scales, 8 neighbors and uniform patterns. As third general purpose method we employ the improved fisher vectors (IFV [14]) computed from SIFT descriptors on a dense 6×6 pixel grid. The fourth method, further denoted as fractal analysis based method (FRAC [16]), was especially developed for the classification of celiac disease and is based on pre-filtering images using the rotation invariant MR8 filterbank, followed by computing the local fractal dimension (see [16]) of the resulting filter responses and applying the bag-of-visual words (BoW) approach to them. We rely on in-house MATLAB implementations for LBP, LTP and FRAC and use the implementation of IFV as provided by *VLFeat*. The comparison methods are classified using SVMs in an analogous manner as for the CNN features.

4.2   Results

The results of our experiments are presented in Table 5. The standard deviations are given in brackets. The best result of each network architecture and classification strategy is given in bold face numbers.

As we can seen in Table 5, the highest CNN results are achieved using the Deep and Very-Deep network architectures combined with large or medium sized filters. Using only 10 filters in the first convolutional layer is insufficient for the classification of celiac disease, but using 48 filters achieves similar results as using 96. The two deeper CNN architectures with large or medium sized filters achieve classification rates of $\approx 90\%$ and hence outperform the comparison methods,

Table 5. Results of the CNNs and comparison methods

Very-shallow networks

Nr. of filters\Size	CNN			CNN &SVM			CNN &SVM &PCA		
	large	medium	small	large	medium	small	large	medium	small
10	85.8(2.3)	85.9(1.7)	86.0(2.0)	89.5(1.9)	88.6(1.9)	91.1(2.9)	89.1(2.1)	88.7(1.6)	91.0(2.7)
48	**88.0**(1.1)	87.4(1.6)	87.6(1.6)	92.5(2.4)	93.3(3.0)	**94.4**(2.9)	92.7(2.7)	93.3(2.7)	**94.3**(3.1)
96	87.5(1.3)	86.8(1.7)	87.9(2.0)	92.1(2.2)	92.8(2.4)	93.3(2.2)	92.2(2.5)	92.6(2.5)	93.3(2.5)

Shallow networks

Nr. of filters\Size	CNN			CNN &SVM			CNN &SVM &PCA		
	large	medium	small	large	medium	small	large	medium	small
10	82.6(4.2)	86.1(2.7)	86.3(1.5)	87.2(2.3)	88.9(1.6)	88.2(2.1)	86.9(2.4)	88.8(1.6)	87.9(2.2)
48	88.5(2.6)	89.9(1.3)	89.1(1.3)	92.1(2.1)	93.3(2.3)	93.2(1.6)	92.0(2.1)	93.3(2.4)	92.9(1.8)
96	88.5(1.4)	**90.0**(1.8)	89.6(1.4)	92.3(2.4)	**94.1**(2.6)	92.9(2.1)	92.4(2.4)	**94.1**(2.4)	93.1(2.2)

Deep networks

Nr. of filters\Size	CNN			CNN &SVM			CNN &SVM &PCA		
	large	medium	small	large	medium	small	large	medium	small
10	87.9(1.4)	89.6(1.4)	88.9(1.2)	93.2(2.6)	92.9(2.1)	92.4(2.1)	93.3(2.6)	93.0(2.2)	92.2(2.2)
48	89.8(1.6)	**90.5**(1.6)	89.8(1.3)	**96.7**(3.0)	96.4(2.8)	95.9(2.4)	**96.6**(3.0)	96.4(2.9)	95.7(2.3)
96	89.1(1.7)	89.9(1.3)	89.4(1.7)	96.5(3.2)	96.4(2.7)	95.4(3.3)	96.5(3.2)	**96.6**(2.6)	95.5(3.0)

Very-deep networks

Nr. of filters\Size	CNN			CNN &SVM			CNN &SVM &PCA		
	large	medium	small	large	medium	small	large	medium	small
10	88.7(1.4)	88.2(2.2)	88.0(1.6)	94.6(2.6)	93.0(2.2)	91.6(2.2)	94.7(2.7)	93.0(2.3)	91.8(2.3)
48	89.5(1.8)	89.3(2.0)	89.2(1.9)	96.5(3.7)	95.7(3.1)	95.6(2.6)	96.5(3.7)	95.7(3.1)	95.5(2.5)
96	**90.3**(1.7)	89.8(1.6)	89.4(1.3)	**97.0**(3.1)	96.5(2.6)	95.4(3.3)	**97.1**(3.4)	96.5(2.6)	95.3(3.1)

Comparison methods

LBP	LTP		IFV			FRAC		
86.4(2.7)	**89.5**(1.8)		84.7(2.8)			80.1(3.9)		

whose highest classification rate is 89.5% (LTP). Combining CNNs and SVMs furtherly improves the results for about 3–7%. Additionally applying PCA to the CNN features has only a minimal effect to the results. The best results (≈97%) are achieved using SVM classification (with or without PCA) applied to the CNN features of the Very-Deep net with 96 filters of size $11 \times 11 \times 3$ in the first convolutional layer.

5   Conclusion

In this work we showed that deep CNN architectures are very suited for the classification of celiac disease based on endoscopic image data. These CNN networks outperform other state-of-the-art image representation approaches. Simpler and more shallow-architectures cannot compete with the deeper architectures. Using large or medium filter dimensions generally leads to higher results than using smaller filter dimensions.

Applying SVMs on the activations of the nets furtherly improves the results of the CNNs for about 3–7% up to a maximum of ≈97%. The highest result was achieved using SVM classification, the deepest architecture (Very-Deep), the largest filter dimension and the highest number of filters (96 filters of size $11 \times 11 \times 3$ in the first convolutional layer).

References

1. Biagi, F., Rondonotti, E., Campanella, J., Villa, F., Bianchi, P.I., Klersy, C., Franchis, R.D., Corazza, G.R.: Video capsule endoscopy and histology for small-bowel mucosa evaluation: a comparison performed by blinded observers. Clin. Gastroenterol. Hepatol. **4**(8), 998–1003 (2006)
2. Chand, N., Mihas, A.A.: Celiac disease: current concepts in diagnosis and treatment. J. Clin. Gastroenterol. **40**(1), 3–14 (2006)
3. Emura, F., Saito, Y.: Narrow-band imaging optical chromocolonoscopy: advantages and limitations. World J. Gastroenterol. **14**(31), 4867–4872 (2008)
4. Fan, R.E., Chang, K.W., Hsieh, C.J., Wang, X.R., Lin, C.J.: Liblinear: a library for large linear classification. J. Mach. Learn. Res. **9**, 1871–1874 (2008)
5. Fasano, A., Berti, I., Gerarduzzi, T., Not, T., Colletti, R.B., Drago, S., Elitsur, Y., Green, P.H.R., Guandalini, S., Hill, I.D., Pietzak, M., Ventura, A., Thorpe, M., Kryszak, D., Fornaroli, F., Wasserman, S.S., Murray, J.A., Horvath, K.: Prevalence of celiac disease in at-risk and not-at-risk groups in the united states: a large multicenter study. Arch. Intern. Med. **163**, 286–292 (2003)
6. Gadermayr, M., Hegenbart, S., Kwitt, R., Uhl, A.: Narrow band imaging versus white-light: what is best for computer-assisted diagnosis of celiac disease? In: Proceedings of the 13th IEEE International Symposium on Biomedical Imaging (ISBI 2016), pp. 355–359, April 2016
7. Gasbarrini, A., Ojetti, V., Cuoco, L., Cammarota, G., Migneco, A., Armuzzi, A., Pola, P., Gasbarrini, G.: Lack of endoscopic visualization of intestinal villi with the immersion technique in overt atrophic celiac disease. Gastrointest. Endosc. **57**, 348–351 (2003)
8. He, K., Zhang, X., Ren, S., Sun, J.: Delving deep into rectifiers: surpassing human-level performance on imagenet classification. In: CoRR (2015)
9. Hegenbart, S., Uhl, A., Vécsei, A.: Survey on computer aided decision support for diagnosis of celiac disease. Comput. Biol. Med. **65**, 348–358 (2015)
10. Jiang, J., Trundle, P., Ren, J.: Medical image analysis with artificial neural networks. Comput. Med. Imaging Graph. **34**(8), 617–631 (2010)
11. Krizhevsky, A., Sutskever, I., Hinton, G.E.: Imagenet classification with deep convolutional neural networks. Adv. Neural Inf. Process. Syst. **25**, 1097–1105 (2012)
12. Niveloni, S., Fiorini, A., Dezi, R., Pedreira, S., Smecuol, E., Vazquez, H., Cabanne, A., Boerr, L.A., Valero, J., Kogan, Z., Maurino, E., Bai, J.C.: Usefulness of video-duodenoscopy and vital dye staining as indicators of mucosal atrophy of celiac disease: assessment of interobserver agreement. Gastrointest. Endosc. **47**(3), 223–229 (1998)
13. Ojala, T., Pietikäinen, M., Harwood, D.: A comparative study of texture measures with classification based on feature distributions. Pattern Recogn. **29**(1), 51–59 (1996)
14. Perronnin, F., Liu, Y., Sanchez, J., Poirier, H.: Large-scale image retrieval with compressed fisher vectors. In: Proceedings of CVPR 2010, pp. 3384–3391 (2010)

15. Tan, X., Triggs, B.: Enhanced local texture feature sets for face recognition under difficult lighting conditions. In: Zhou, S.K., Zhao, W., Tang, X., Gong, S. (eds.) AMFG 2007. LNCS, vol. 4778, pp. 168–182. Springer, Heidelberg (2007). doi:10. 1007/978-3-540-75690-3_13

16. Uhl, A., Vécsei, A., Wimmer, G.: Fractal analysis for the viewpoint invariant classification of celiac disease. In: Proceedings of the 7th International Symposium on Image and Signal Processing (ISPA 2011), Dubrovnik, Croatia, pp. 727–732, September 2011

17. Valitutti, F., Oliva, S., Iorfida, D., Aloi, M., Gatti, S., Trovato, C.M., Montuori, M., Tiberti, A., Cucchiara, S., Di Nardo, G.: Narrow band imaging combined with water immersion technique in the diagnosis of celiac disease. Dig. Liver Dis. **46**(12), 1099–1102 (2014)

18. Vedaldi, A., Lenc, K.: Matconvnet - convolutional neural networks for matlab. In: Proceeding of the ACM International Conference on Multimedia, pp. 689–692 (2015)

19. Yu, J., Chen, J., Xiang, Z.Q., Zou, Y.X.: A hybrid convolutional neural networks with extreme learning machine for wce image classification. In: IEEE International Conference on Robotics and Biomimetics (ROBIO) 2015, pp. 1822–1827, December 2015

20. Zhu, R., Zhang, R., Xue, D.: Lesion detection of endoscopy images based on convolutional neural network features. In: 8th International Congress on Image and Signal Processing (CISP), pp. 372–376, October 2015

21. Zou, Y., Li, L., Wang, Y., Yu, J., Li, Y., Deng, W.J.: Classifying digestive organs in wireless capsule endoscopy images based on deep convolutional neural network. IEEE Int. Conf. Digit. Signal Process. (DSP) **2015**, 1274–1278 (2015)

A System for Augmented Reality Guided Laparoscopic Tumour Resection with Quantitative Ex-vivo User Evaluation

Toby Collins[1]([⊠]), Pauline Chauvet[1], Clément Debize[1], Daniel Pizarro[1,2], Adrien Bartoli[1], Michel Canis[1], and Nicolas Bourdel[1]

[1] ALCoV-ISIT, UMR 6284 CNRS/Université d'Auvergne, Clermont-Ferrand, France
Toby.Collins@gmail.com
[2] Geintra Research Group, Universidad de Alcalá, Alcalá de Henares, Spain

Abstract. Augmented Reality (AR) guidance systems are currently being developed to help laparoscopic surgeons locate hidden structures such as tumours and major vessels. This can be achieved by registering pre-operative 3D data such as CT or MRI with the laparoscope's live video. For soft organs this is very challenging, and quantitative evaluation is both difficult and limited in the literature. It has been done previously by measuring registration accuracy using retrospective (non-live) data. However a performance evaluation of a real-time system in live use has not been presented. The clinical benefit has therefore not been measured. We describe an AR guidance system based on an existing one with several important improvements, that has been evaluated in an ex-vivo pre-clinical study for guiding tumour resections with porcine kidneys. The main improvement is a considerably better way to visually guide the surgeon, by showing them how to access the tumour with an incision tool. We call this *Tool Access Visualisation*. Performance was measured with the negative margin rate across 59 resected pseudo-tumours. This was 85.2% with AR guidance and 41.9% without, showing a very significant improvement ($p = 0.0010$, two-tailed Fisher's exact test).

1 Introduction and Background

There is much ongoing research to develop AR guidance systems to improve laparosurgery. One important goal is to visualise hidden internal structures such as tumours and major vessels by augmenting optical images from a laparoscope with pre-operative 3D radiological data from MRI or CT. Despite considerable research, robust systems capable of handling soft tissue deformation do not yet exist. To achieve this three main challenges must be overcome. The first is to build a segmented deformable model of the organ and its internal structures from the radiological data. This process is the least time-critical because it can be done before intervention. The second challenge is real-time registration, where the goal is to transform the model to the laparoscope's coordinate frame using live visual information present in the laparoscope's image. The third challenge is visualisation, where the goal is to augment the laparoscope's image with data

T. Peters et al. (Eds.): CARE 2016, LNCS 10170, pp. 114–126, 2017.
DOI: 10.1007/978-3-319-54057-3_11

from the organ model in order to guide the surgeon. This paper focuses on the registration and visualisation problems, for which a number of approaches have been proposed. Registration algorithms have been described and tested with various organs including the liver [6,7,11], uterus [3,4] and kidney [9,12,13]. To date most previous approaches have been developed for robotic surgery with stereo laparoscopes. However there are a few that work with monocular laparoscopes [3,4,6,9,12]. The challenges with monocular laparoscopes are far greater due to the lack of depth information. However they are used in the majority of laparosurgery due to several factors including cost, image resolution and smaller port size. Of these, the systems which are capable of robust registration over long durations are [4,12]. These work by first performing an initial registration, to align the model to one [12] or several [4] reference laparoscopic images. Then 2D texture features are detected in the reference images with *e.g.* SURF [2] and mapped onto the model's surface. Once done the model is automatically registered to new laparoscopic images using feature-based tracking. An important difference between [4,12] is that in [12] the initial registration was done manually with a rigid model, whereas in [4] it was done semi-automatically with a deformable model. Therefore [4] could handle deformation due to insufflation and other factors, which is required for accurate registration of soft organs.

A main shortcoming of the above approaches is the lack of thorough quantitative evaluation, and the lack of live usage tests. In the above papers all quantitative results were presented using retrospective videos from pre-recorded surgeries. Therefore evaluating the practical benefit of the system for surgical guidance was not done. From a technical standpoint, moving from pre-recorded videos to live surgery is far from trivial. The main issues are time constraints: any time for manual stages becomes significant and parameter tuning is not really possible. Furthermore, when processing live videos the effective frame-rate is limited by the AR system's speed, which is usually well below the frame-rate of a pre-recorded video (typically 30–50 fps). Therefore inter-frame motion is more significant, and depending on the algorithm can severely affect performance.

We present an AR guidance system with monocular laparoscopes, based on [4], which runs in real-time and which has been tested live with a systematic preclinical user study. This evaluation measured the benefit of AR guided tumour resection using ex-vivo porcine kidneys. To achieve this a number of improvements were made to [4]. These were for generalising the approach to general biomechanical organ models, reducing manual processing time and a much better approach to AR visualisation, which we call *Tool Access Visualisation*.

2   AR Guidance System

We first describe the system's inputs (Sect. 2.1) and give a global overview of the registration algorithm (Sect. 2.2). We then describe the two main components of the registration algorithm, which are the *initial registration* and *tracking* stages (Sects. 2.3 and 2.4 respectively). Lastly we present Tool Access Visualisation (Sect. 2.5).

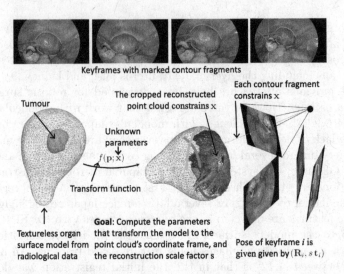

Fig. 1. The initial registration problem illustrated with a human uterus. Four keyframes are shown in the first row with their associated contour fragments.

2.1   System Inputs

The system requires a segmented pre-operative biomechanical 3D model, which has surface meshes for the organ and internal structures that are to be visualised. Here the internal structures are tumours and their *safe tissue margin*. A safe tissue margin is a border around the tumour of healthy tissue which should also be removed, whose thickness w depends on the risk factor of the particular tumour. We require two functions from the biomechanical model. The first is the *transform function* $f(\mathbf{p}; \mathbf{x}_t) : \Omega \to \mathbb{R}^3$, which transforms a 3D point $\mathbf{p}$ in the model's 3D domain $\Omega \subset \mathbb{R}^3$ to the laparoscope's coordinates frame, where the vector $\mathbf{x}_t$ denotes the model's parameters at time t. The second is an internal energy function $E_{internal}(\mathbf{x}_t) : \mathbb{R}^d \to \mathbb{R}^+$ which gives the internal energy for transforming the organ with $\mathbf{x}_t$, where d is the dimensionality of $\mathbf{x}_t$. Both f and $E_{internal}$ must be continuous and at least first-order differentiable. We also require the laparoscope to be intrinsically calibrated.

We describe here the input models used in the presented experiments to make things concrete for the reader. These came from T2 weighted MRI with segmentation done semi-automatically using MITK [14]. The deformation models were tetrahedral Finite Element Models (FEMs) built with a 3D vertex grid (6 mm spacing) cropped to the organ. Therefore $\mathbf{x}_t$ held the unknown 3D positions of the FEM's vertices in laparoscope coordinates. Trilinear interpolation was used to compute $f(\mathbf{p}; \mathbf{x}_t)$. For $E_{internal}$ the Saint Venant-Kirchoff strain energy was used, with rough generic values for the Young's modulus E and Poisson's ratio ν. These were for healthy kidney tissue $E = 7\,\mathrm{kPa}$, $\nu = 0.43$ [5], healthy uterus tissue $E = 96\,\mathrm{kPa}$, $\nu = 0.45$ [10] and myomas $E = 532\,\mathrm{kPa}$, $\nu = 0.48$ [10]. Note that in the registration problem there is always a balancing weight between the internal energy and energy coming from image cues (which have no real physical meaning). Therefore only the relative values of E are important to us (with respect to the balancing weight), rather than their absolute values.

2.2   Overview of the Registration Algorithm

The registration problem is to determine $\mathbf{x}_t$ for a given live laparoscopic image streamed at time t. We break this down into two stages. The first is a non-live stage which is called the *initial registration stage*. The second is a live-stage which is called the *tracking stage*. The purpose of the initial registration stage is two-fold. Firstly, it is to determine the change of shape of the organ between its pre-operative state and an intra-operative reference state. Secondly, it is used to associate texture with the organ's surface, which is required in the tracking stage. To achieve high robustness we make a simplifying assumption in the tracking stage, which is that the organ does not deform significantly during this stage. Therefore the tracking stage can be modelled with *rigid update transforms*, which can be estimated far more quickly and robustly than deformable transforms. In practice this assumption is reasonable by asking the surgeon to not physically deform the organ during the tracking stage (*i.e.* the period that they wish to use live AR guidance). Formally, the two stages break down $f(\mathbf{p}; \mathbf{x}_t)$ as $f(\mathbf{p}; \mathbf{x}_t) = M(f(\mathbf{p}; \mathbf{x}); \mathbf{R}_t, \mathbf{t}_t)$. Here $\mathbf{x}$ denotes the organ's interventional reference state. The function $M(\cdot; \mathbf{R}_t, \mathbf{t}_t) : \mathbb{R}^3 \to \mathbb{R}^3$ denotes a rigid update transform at time t, parameterised by a rotation $\mathbf{R}_t \in \mathcal{SO}_3$ and translation $\mathbf{t}_t \in \mathbb{R}^3$. Thus the initial registration stage is for estimating $\mathbf{x}$ and the tracking stage is for estimating $(\mathbf{R}_t, \mathbf{t}_t)$. To have live AR, only the tracking stage needs to be real-time. The time to solve the initial registration stage is a delay period before AR can run. With our current implementation this takes approximately three minutes with non-optimised C++/Matlab code on a standard workstation PC (approximately two minutes for manual pre-processing and one minute for optimisation). The tracking stage is an implementation of [3] in optimised C++/CUDA and runs at approximately 16 fps.

2.3   The Initial Registration Stage

Overview. We illustrate the problem setup in Fig. 1 using a human uterus with a deep myoma. This stage is more challenging to solve than the tracking stage because *(i)* we have no texture information associated with the organ's surface (because it comes from a radiological image segmentation), and *(ii)* it is a deformable registration. We tackle it similarly to [4] using a 3D point cloud reconstruction of the interventional scene by running rigid Structure-from-Motion (SfM), for which mature methods exist. To do this we require some sample images of the organ, known as *keyframes*, observing it from different viewpoints and distances. In our experiments typically no more than 10 are required, which are gathered as the surgeon performs an initial exploration of the organ (referred to as the *exploratory phase*). Note that a SfM reconstruction is up to an unknown global scale factor s. We resolve this jointly with registration.

We formulate the problem as a non-linear energy-minimisation problem, with energies coming from prior and data terms. The prior term encodes the model's internal energy, which is used to regularise the problem. The data terms are illustrate in Fig. 1. The first involves the point cloud reconstruction, and encourages the organ's surface mesh to fit to the point cloud. Importantly, this is a *robust* data term, which accounts for the fact that the reconstruction may contain outliers or some residual background and/or occluding structures. The second data term complements the first and uses contour cues. Specifically, it is a silhouette contour term which makes the organ model's silhouette align to its associated contours in the keyframe images. This is complementary to the point cloud data term for two reasons. Firstly, we never usually reconstruct points reliably at these regions due to occlusions. Secondly, it anchors the organ's silhouette to the contour fragments, which is a strong constraint. We implement this data term with some manual assistance, similarly to [4]. Specifically, a human operator marks in a keyframe where they can confidently see the organ's silhouette contours (Fig. 1, first row). We call these *contour fragments*. The operator does not need to mark contour fragments in all keyframes (it can be done with only one). If more keyframes are marked then we have more constraints, but it takes more time. We use a default of four keyframes. They also do not need to be contiguous. Optionally, an anatomical landmark data term can also be included [4], which is used to align distinct landmarks that can be found on the organ's surface in the pre-operative and laparoscopic images. In [4] for the uterus, these were the Fallopian tube/uterus junctions, which were manually located. Landmarks help guide registration if the initialisation is poor or there is very strong deformation. In the presented experiments we do not use them in the optimisation process, so are omitted from the energy function.

The main improvements over [4] are summarised as follows:

- In [4] the deformable model used was a 3D affine model. This was shown to be sufficient for simple deformations of the human uterus but is not sufficient in general. We extend the approach to work with general biomechanical models. This requires changing the core energy function to include the model's internal energy (without this the problem is highly under-constrained), and to correct the interventional reconstruction's scale factor s. Note that in [4], s could be absorbed into the affine model's coefficients. This is generally not possible with biomechanical models because a change of scale affects the internal energy.
- In [4] the organ's surface was assumed to have disc topology. We generalise this to arbitrary fixed topologies.
- We have sped up the process of marking contour fragments considerably with a touch-screen interface, where the operator marks them with rough finger strokes. These strokes then guide an automatic refinement method based on intelligent scissors [8]. This reduces manual effort, typically taking less than 10 s for a single keyframe.

Interventional 3D reconstruction. During the exploratory phase the laparoscopic video is saved to disk, then N keyframes $\{K_1, \dots K_N\}$ are extracted. We index these with $i \in [1, N]$. This is done by uniformly sampling the video into N intervals with a default $N = 12$. For each interval i we take the keyframe K_i to be the one with the lowest optical motion, using the Sum-of-Absolute Difference (SAD) as the metric computed between consecutive frame pairs. This is done to improve the quality of the reconstruction because SfM work best with sharper images. We then run a state-of-the-art dense SfM algorithm (currently Photoscan [1]) to compute a dense point cloud reconstruction $\mathcal{Q} \stackrel{\text{def}}{=} \{\mathbf{q}_1, \dots \mathbf{q}_M\}$, $\mathbf{q}_j \in \mathbb{R}^3$, and the keyframe camera pose matrices $\mathbf{M}_i \in \mathcal{SE}_4$. These hold the laparoscope's rotation matrix $\mathbf{R}_i \in \mathcal{SO}_3$ and translation vector $\mathbf{t}_i \in \mathbb{R}^3$ relative to the point cloud. Recall that $\mathcal{Q}$ and $\mathbf{t}_i$ are defined up to the unknown scale factor $s \in \mathbb{R}^+$. We chose Photoscan because it has been shown to work well on laparoscopic data [3] and can produce far denser reconstructions than purely feature-based methods. There may exist some keyframes whose pose is not computable, due to e.g. insufficient visual overlap. We currently deal with this by simply removing the keyframe. The point cloud $\mathcal{Q}$ may contain background and/or foreground structures that partially occlude the organ. We currently deal with this by a human operator cropping them using a fast lasso-based user interface [1]. To reduce time we do not require the cropping to be perfect. We allow some non-organ points to remain in $\mathcal{Q}$ and we deal with them by making the associated data term robust (see below). In some instances SfM may fail, which typically occurs when the keyframe overlap is insufficient. This can usually be resolved by extracting more keyframes by doubling the number of intervals and re-running SfM. In rare events SfM may still fail, due to very weak texture. In these cases we find image enhancement such as Storz's CLARA can help. Alternatively, SLAM could be tried because unlike SfM it exploits temporal continuity.

Initialisation. We initialise $\mathbf{x}$ with a rigid transform, denoted by $\mathbf{M} \in \mathcal{SE}_4$. In some cases $\mathbf{M}$ can be considered known *a priori*, for example if the laparoscope is assumed to be in a canonical position. When this cannot be assumed, we compute it with a small amount of manual interaction as follows. A small number of point correspondences (at least four) are selected on the organ's surface model and one of the keyframe images. Without loss of generality let this be the first keyframe K_1. We then compute a rigid transform $\mathbf{M}_a$ from model coordinates to laparoscope coordinates, by fitting the correspondences using OpenCV's PnP method. The point correspondences are computed using an interactive user interface, where the model can be freely rotated to present it from a similar viewpoint as the keyframe's viewpoint. This significantly eases the operator's task. We then initialise s as follows. First we transform the model by $\mathbf{M}_a$ and render it using OpenGL with the same intrinsic parameters as the laparoscope. This generates a depth map $d(x, y)$, and we compute s by comparing depths in d to the depths of $\mathcal{Q}$. Specifically, let $\tilde{d}_j$ be the depth of $\mathbf{q}_j$ to the laparoscope in keyframe 1, and (x_j, y_j) be its 2D position in the keyframe's image. We can then estimate s by $s \approx d(x_j, y_j)/\tilde{d}_j$. Note that only points that project within the render's silhouette can be used. To compute s robustly, we compute it as the median value from all such points. Finally, the transform $\mathbf{M}$ is given by the composition $\mathbf{M} = \mathbf{M}_s \mathbf{M}_i^{-1} \mathbf{M}_s^{-1} \mathbf{M}_a$, where $\mathbf{M}_s$ is an isotropic scaling by s.

The energy function. To improve clarity we define all image points in normalised pixel coordinates, which is possible given the intrinsic calibration. The energy function $E(\mathbf{x}, s) \in \mathbb{R}^+$ consists of the point cloud data term E_{point}, which encourages the organ's surface to fit to $\mathcal{Q}$, the contour data tern $E_{contour}$, which encourages the organ's silhouette contours to fit to the contour fragments, and the prior term, which is the model's internal energy $E_{internal}(\mathbf{x})$:

$$E(\mathbf{x}, s) = E_{point}(\mathbf{x}, s; \mathcal{Q}) + \lambda_{contour} E_{contour}(\mathbf{x}, s; \mathcal{C}_1, \ldots, \mathcal{C}_N) + \lambda_{internal} E_{internal}(\mathbf{x}) \quad (1)$$

where $\lambda_{contour}$ and $\lambda_{internal}$ are scalar weights specific to the organ category. The set $\mathcal{C}_i$ denotes all pixels on the contour fragments in keyframe i.

We construct E_{point} using an Iterative Closest Point (ICP)-based energy. This works using a set of *virtual point correspondences* $\mathcal{P} = \{\mathbf{p}_1, \ldots \mathbf{p}_M\}$ with $\mathbf{p}_j \in \partial\Omega$ denoting the unknown position of point j on the organ's surface mesh. For a given $(\mathbf{x}, s)$ we compute E_{point} as follows. First we transform the organ's surface mesh according to $f(\cdot; \mathbf{x})$ and rescale the point cloud with $\hat{\mathbf{q}}_j \leftarrow s\,\mathbf{q}_j$. We then set $\mathbf{p}_j$ as the closest point to $\hat{\mathbf{q}}_j$ on the surface's mesh. We define E_{point} using a robust point-to-plane distance function, which is inspired by point-to-plane ICP with rigid objects. This allows the model to slide over the point cloud without resistance, and is defined as follows:

$$E_{point}(\mathbf{x}, s; \mathcal{Q}) = \frac{1}{M} \sum_{j=1}^{M} \rho\left(d_{plane}\left(v_j(\mathbf{x}), \hat{\mathbf{q}}_j\right)\right) \quad (2)$$

The function $v_j(\mathbf{x}) \in \mathbb{R}^4$ gives the organ surface's tangent plane at $f(\mathbf{p}_j)$. The function $d_{plane}(\mathbf{v}, \mathbf{q})$ gives the signed distance between a plane $\mathbf{v}$ and a 3D point $\mathbf{q}$. The function $\rho : \mathbb{R} \to \mathbb{R}^+$ is an *M-estimator* and is crucial to achieve robust registration. Its purpose is to align the reconstructed point $\hat{\mathbf{q}}_j$ with the organ's surface, but to do so robustly to account for non-organ points being in $\mathcal{Q}$ or poorly reconstructed points. The model should not align these points, and the M-estimator facilitates this by reducing the influence of their alignment error on E. We have tested various types and good results are obtained with pseudo-L1 $\rho(x) \stackrel{\text{def}}{=} \sqrt{x^2 + \epsilon}$ with $\epsilon = 10^{-3}$ being a small constant, which is used to make ρ differentiable everywhere.

We construct $E_{contour}$ similarly with virtual point correspondences. Specifically, for a given pair $(\mathbf{x}, s)$ and a given keyframe i we construct a set of virtual correspondences $\mathcal{R}_i = \{\mathbf{r}_1, \ldots, \mathbf{r}_{C(i)}\}$ where $\mathbf{r}_k \in \partial\Omega$ denotes the unknown position of the kth contour fragment pixel $\mathbf{c}_k$ on the model's surface. The virtual correspondences are points on the organ surface mesh's occluding contours, and are computed as follows. First we transform the organ's surface mesh according to $f(\cdot; \mathbf{x})$, then transform it to laparoscope coordinates using $(\mathbf{R}_i, s\,\mathbf{t}_i)$. We then render the surface mesh using OpenGL, using the same intrinsic parameters as the laparoscope. We then take the render's silhouette and extract all the pixels on the render's boundary, which is put into a set $\mathcal{B}$. For each contour fragment pixel $\mathbf{c}_k \in \mathcal{C}_j$ we compute its closest point $\mathbf{b}_k \in \mathcal{B}$ and form a correspondence with it. We then compute the 3D position of $\mathbf{b}_k$ in model coordinates, which is easy to do with an OpenGL shader, and assign it to $\mathbf{r}_k$. We then evaluate $E_{contour}$ as the alignment error from all correspondences:

$$E_{contour}(\mathbf{x}, s; \mathcal{C}_1, \ldots, \mathcal{C}_N) = \frac{1}{C} \sum_{i=1}^{N} \sum_{(\mathbf{c}_k \in \mathcal{C}_i, \mathbf{r}_k \in \mathcal{R}_i)} \rho(\|\pi(f(\mathbf{r}_k)) - \mathbf{c}_k\|_2) \quad (3)$$

where $\pi([x, y, z]^\top) \overset{\text{def}}{=} 1/z[x, y]^\top$ is the perspective projection function and C is the total number of contour fragment pixels. Here the M-estimator ρ is also used to handle the fact that some of the contour fragment pixels may be erroneous, which can sometimes occur if the intelligent scissoring fails to snap correctly at low-contrast edges.

Optimisation. We optimise E by iterative non-linear optimization using a stiff-to-flexible strategy. This is used to improve convergence by starting with a stiff model, optimising E, then reducing the stiffness to account for more and more deformation. We use a default of $l = 6$ stiffness levels with $\lambda_{internal}(l) = 2\lambda_{internal}(l-1)$. For each level we alternate between computing the virtual correspondence sets ($\mathcal{R}_i$ and $\mathcal{P}$) and optimising E, which is done with a Gauss-Newton iteration and backtracking line search. This continues until either convergence is reached or 10 iterations have passed. At the final stiffness level we optimize until convergence. Convergence however is not guaranteed because of the point-to-plane distance function in E_{point}. Specifically, the energy may increase after $\mathcal{P}$ is re-computed. We handle this by using the point-to-point distance at the final level, because this ensures E will decrease at each iteration.

2.4   The Tracking Stage

Having solved the initial registration we initiate the tracking stage, which updates the initial registration in real-time using live images streamed from the laparoscope. We solve this with an existing feature-based method [3]. This works by first extracting 2D features in the keyframe images, then matching them with RANSAC-based rigid registration to each new image. The advantages of [3] are it is robust to occlusions from *e.g.* surgical tools, handles partial views and viewpoint changes. Unlike SLAM-based tracking methods it does not use frame-to-frame tracking. Instead it performs *tracking-by-detection*. This allows it to register over long durations and can trivially recover when the organ is not visible for certain periods, such as when the surgeon removes and then reinserts the laparoscope or cleans the lens. In cases when the organ is assumed to be fixed relative to background structures, we can track using features from both the organ and background structures. This improves stability if the organ's texture is weak, and we do this in the ex-vivo user study.

2.5   AR Guidance with Tool Access Visualisation

Having registered, the final task is AR visualisation. We briefly describe *Transparent Blending* (TB) visualisation, which is the previous approach used with

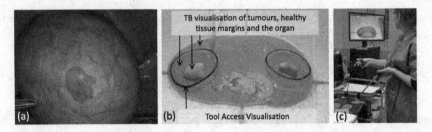

Fig. 2. (a) AR with Transparent Blending (TB) visualisation taken from [4]. (b) Our AR visualisation combining Transparent Blending with Tool Access Visualisation. (c) Our AR system in live operation during the ex-vivo user study.

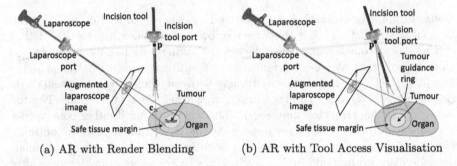

(a) AR with Render Blending   (b) AR with Tool Access Visualisation

Fig. 3. The difference between typical AR visualisation of a tumour (a), which does not take into account the position and access direction of the incision tool, and the proposed Tool Access Visualisation (b) which does.

monocular laparoscopes. It works by first rendering the tumours on the laparoscope's image plane, then a composite image is made by blending the render with the real image to give the impression the organ is transparent. An example from [4] is shown in Fig. 2(a) where two myomas are visualised with TB. TB however has a serious limitation which has not been previously addressed, and we find it can actually *mis-guide the surgeon*. The problem is illustrated in Fig. 3(a) and is as follows. When a surgeon actually uses TB to resect a tumour they usually assume it indicates where they should cut to access the tumour. This however is incorrect. It just shows the position of the tumour from the viewpoint of the laparoscope. Often they assume the tumour's centre would be reached by cutting into the organ from the rendered tumour's centre $c \in \mathbb{R}^2$. This is not the case as shown in Fig. 3(a). In our user study we found this is a significant problem with smaller and/or deeper tumours, and can cause them to be missed.

What the surgeon actually wants is to be shown how to reach the tumour using the incision tool. Furthermore, surgeons typically want to also see the tumour's safe tissue margin. We provide both information with what we call *Tool Access Visualisation*, which is shown in Fig. 2(b). Its associated geometry is shown in Fig. 3(b). Tool Access Visualisation works by showing the tumour's safe tissue margin projected onto the organ's surface as a ring, which we call the *tumour guidance ring*. The idea is that if the surgeon were to cut into the organ along the guidance ring, they would segment the tumour with a minimal margin of w mm. At present we do not visualise uncertainty in the margin's location, which is important for real clinical use, and leave this to future work.

We achieve Tool Access Visualisation with *two* projections. The first is a perspective projection of the margin's surface onto the organ's surface, using a centre-of-projection located at the incision tool's port centre $\mathbf{p} \in \mathbb{R}^3$. The second is a perspective projection of the projected margin's perimeter onto the laparoscope's optical image (shown as rings in Fig. 2(b)). To achieve this we need to know $\mathbf{p}$. Recall that the organ has been registered in laparoscope coordinates, therefore we need $\mathbf{p}$ in laparoscope coordinates. It may be possible to estimate $\mathbf{p}$ automatically using external and/or internal tool tracking, however this is left to future work. Here we assume $\mathbf{p}$ is given *a priori*. In our user study, where the ports are located on a pelvic trainer, this is simple and can be done offline by taking physical measurements. We complete the visualisation by combining Tool Access Visualisation with TB visualisation (Fig. 2(b)) to show tumours (solid fill), organ (wireframe) and safe tissue margins (wireframe).

3   Evaluation

This section is divided into two parts. The first is the main part describing our ex-vivo user study. The second part shows our system doing live in-vivo registration of a porcine kidney during a laparoscopic training exercise. All the procedures were performed in the operating room of the International Centre of Endoscopic Surgery (CICE), France, approval number C63 18 113.

3.1   Ex-vivo User Study Evaluation

We used 29 porcine kidneys recovered from pigs operated after resident training. For each kidney pseudo-tumours were created by injecting alginate, a hardening hydrocolloid, of between 4 mm and 10 mm in diameter. In total 59 pseudo-tumours were injected at arbitrary sub-surface positions, with an average of 2.5 per kidney. We used safe tissue margins of 5 mm. Kidney models were made as described in Sect. 2.1 from 3T MRI images (0.4 mm resolution and slice thickness 1.5 mm). The interventional equipment is shown in Fig. 2(c) and consisted of a Karl Storz 10 mm laparoscope column with CLARA image enhancement, a surgical grasper, an incision tool, a laparoscopic pelvic trainer and an instrument with a surgical marker pen attached at the tip (referred to as the *marker instrument*). The AR software ran on a mid-range Intel i7 desktop workstation with an NVidia 980 Ti GPU, with visualisations shown on a 26 inch monitor. Laparosurgery was performed by a skilled final-year resident. The resident spent time training before evaluation to familiarise the task, the guidance software and to provide feedback to improve visualisation. In total 28 pseudo-tumours were resected during this time.

3.2   Interventional Protocol and Equipment

Laparosurgery was performed using the pelvic trainer, with the kidney inserted on a ground surface and the laparoscope and instruments inserted through three ports. The same port configuration was used in all cases. The surgeon was tasked to remove each tumour by cutting out a conic tissue section which included the tumour and its safe tissue margin. The kidneys were divided into two groups (non-randomised): the *AR group* and the *Non-AR group*, with 13 kidneys in the AR group with 29 tumours, and 19 kidneys in the Non-AR group with 33 tumours. Kidneys in the AR group were operated with the AR guidance system activated. Recall that the guidance system is not designed to handle significant deformation or topology change after the initial registration, which occurs when a tumour is resected. This was dealt with in the protocol by having the surgeon first mark dots along the tumour guidance ring using the marker instrument, guided by the AR visualisation. Once completed they used the marks to guide the resection with AR disactivated. For the Non-AR group, the surgeon first consulted the MRI using interactive slice-based visualisation [14]. The task was then performed without AR guidance using the same safe tissue margin of 5 mm.

3.3   Results

We present results with the negative margin rate. A negative margin occurs when the tumour is contained entirely within the resected tissue. A positive margin occurs when either the tumour is completely absent from the resected tissue (a *complete miss*), or if it is partially contained (a *contact*). For three tumours the protocol was not completed properly (the conic section did not cut fully through the kidney) and were excluded. There were 13 negative margins in the Non-AR group (41.9%), with 4 complete misses and 14 contacts. There were 23 negative margins in the AR group (85.2%), with 0 complete misses and 4 contacts. Statistical significance was measured with Fisher's exact two-tailed test with $p = 0.0010$. Therefore the user study indicates a very significant benefit for using the AR guidance system.

3.4   Live In-vivo Registration of a Porcine Kidney

We finish by showing our system in live use for registering *in-vivo* a porcine kidney during a laparoscopic training exercise (Fig. 4). The kidney did not contain a tumour and no ground truth information was available, so the results are merely to demonstrate that the registration system works live and *in-vivo*. The biomechanical kidney model was build as described in Sect. 2.1. The same Storz laparoscope column was used as the user study. An exploratory video was captured lasting approximately 30 s. We show sample keyframes in Fig. 4(b–d) with contour fragments overlaid. Note that only the kidney's upper silhouette contours are visible, with the lower ones being occluded by intestine and peritoneum, which is why there are no contour fragments on the lower half. In Fig. 4(e) we overlay the registered model's surface onto one of the keyframes,

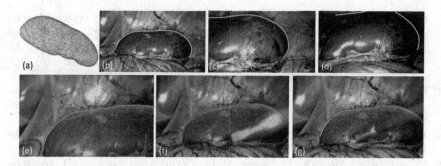

Fig. 4. Live *in-vivo* registration of a porcine kidney. (a) the organ model's surface mesh. (b–d) contour fragments in three keyframes. (e) the surface mesh overlaid on a keyframe after the initial registration with its silhouette contours in red. (f–g) Snapshots of the surface mesh during live tracking, with ground-truth silhouette contours shown in green. Note that the kidney's lower portion is occluded by intestine and peritoneum. Best viewed in colour. (Color figure online)

showing the upper contours aligning well with the image. In Fig. 4(f,g) we show frames from the live tracking stage, which shows robustness to tool occlusions and mild deformations.

4   Conclusion

We have presented a complete system for AR guided laparoscopic tumour resection, and a quantitative ex-vivo user study to measure its benefit in live use, which is the first of its kind. The system has been based on [4] with several major improvements. These include supporting general biomechanical models as inputs, less manual processing and a new visualisation method, called Tool Access Visualisation (TAV), which shows the surgeon how to access a tumour and its safe tissue margin with an incision tool. In future work we aim to conduct a similar user study *in-vivo*, and to test with stereo laparoscopic images, where the point cloud reconstruction would come from stereo triangulation. We also aim to extend Tool Access visualisation to handle non-straight incision tools, such as articulated ones used in robotic laparosurgery.

Acknowledgements. This research was funded by the EU FP7 ERC research grant 307483 FLEXABLE and Almerys Corporation.

References

1. Agisoft photoscan. http://www.agisoft.com. Accessed 07 Feb 2016
2. Bay, H., Ess, A., Tuytelaars, T., Van Gool, L.: Speeded-up robust features (SURF). Comput. Vis. Image Underst. **110**(3), 346–359 (2008)

3. Collins, T., Pizarro, D., Bartoli, A., Canis, M., Bourdel, N.: Realtime wide-baseline registration of the uterus in laparoscopic videos using multiple texture maps. In: Liao, H., Linte, C.A., Masamune, K., Peters, T.M., Zheng, G. (eds.) AE-CAI/MIAR -2013. LNCS, vol. 8090, pp. 162–171. Springer, Heidelberg (2013). doi:10.1007/978-3-642-40843-4_18
4. Collins, T., Pizarro, D., Bartoli, A., Canis, M., Bourdel, N.: Computer-assisted laparoscopic myomectomy by augmenting the uterus with pre-operative MRI data. In: ISMAR (2014)
5. Egorov, V., Tsyuryupa, S., Kanilo, S., Kogit, M., Sarvazyan, A.: Soft tissue elastometer. Med. Eng. Phys. **30**, 206–212 (2008)
6. Haouchine, N., Dequidt, J., Berger, M.-O., Cotin, S.: Monocular 3D reconstruction and augmentation of elastic surfaces with self-occlusion handling. Trans. Vis. Comput. Graph., 14 (2015)
7. Haouchine, N., Dequidt, J., Peterlik, I., Kerrien, E., Berger, M.-O., Cotin, S.: Image-guided simulation of heterogeneous tissue deformation for augmented reality during hepatic surgery. In: ISMAR (2013)
8. Mortensen, E.N., Barrett, W.A.: Intelligent scissors for image composition. In: SIGGRAPH, pp. 191–198 (1995)
9. Nosrati, M.S., Peyrat, J.-M., Abinahed, J., Al-Alao, O., Al-Ansari, A., Abugharbieh, R., Hamarneh, G.: Simultaneous multi-structure segmentation and 3D non-rigid pose estimation in image guided robotic surgery. Trans. Med. Imaging **35**(1), 1–12 (2016)
10. Pearsall, G., Roberts, V.: Passive mechanical properties of uterine muscle (myometrium) tested in vitro. J. Biomech. **4**(11), 167–176 (1978)
11. Plantefève, R., Peterlik, I., Haouchine, N., Cotin, S.: Patient-specific biomechanical modeling for guidance during minimally-invasive hepatic surgery. Ann. Biomed. Eng. (2015)
12. Puerto-Souza, G., Cadeddu, J.A., Mariottini, G.: Toward long-term and accurate AR for monocular endoscopic videos. Biomed. Eng. (2014)
13. Su, L.-M., Vagvolgyi, B.P., Agarwal, R., Reiley, C.E., Taylor, R.H., Hager, G.D.: Augmented reality during robot-assisted laparoscopic partial nephrectomy: toward real-time 3D-CT to stereoscopic video registration. Urology **73**, 896–900 (2009)
14. Wolf, I., Vetter, M., Wegner, I., Nolden, M., Böttger, T., Hastenteufel, M., Schöbinger, M., Kunert, T., Meinzer, H.-P.: The medical imaging interaction toolkit (MITK). http://www.mitk.org/

Author Index

Printed in the United States
By Bookmasters